# Bollywood Abs

## by NEIL FROST

The 12 Week Workout & Diet Plan to Get that LEAN 'SIX PACK' BODY!

## Disclaimer

The Bollywood Abs Program is intended for healthy adults over 16 years of age. This book is for informational and educational purposes and is not medical advice. Always consult a medical or health professional before beginning any exercise or nutrition program. Use of the program, advice, and information contained in this book is at the sole choice and risk of the reader.

## www.bollywood-abs.com

# About Neil Frost

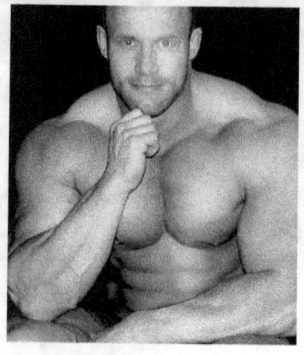 Neil Frost is a successful entrepreneur, fitness company owner and author of the best selling book 'Abs for Life'. Neil has personally mentored many clients from the world of Film, Television, Sport and Music and also many executives from Blue Chip Companies around the world. To date his company SPN Fitness has helped over 10,000 men and women from all walks of life successfully reach their fitness goals.

Neil believes anyone can change their body if they have the willpower. He says "Getting in shape takes time, dedication and sacrifice, it's not a sprint, it's a marathon. It's also a new way of life and one that will take your body to the next level if you stay committed and keep focused"

When asked why he wrote Bollywood Abs, Neil said "I had received literally hundreds and hundreds of emails from Indian men and women who wanted to achieve that six pack body, but where so confused how they could do it with a diet that is typically high in fat, so I took on the challenge of creating a Program and Diet Plan that would include healthy, low fat options of all the Indian favorites, but also include a comprehensive system that will deliver results with even the most basic equipment. I really think Bollywood Abs is the first of its kind."

# CONTENTS

# ACKNOWLEDGEMENTS

I knew when I was going to write this book that there was so much I needed to find out about India itself, its people, its traditions, its diet and its love for fitness and exercise. I couldn't have written this book if I had not actually seen all the above first hand, hence why I travelled to India to write much of this book.

Whilst there I met some truly fantastic people, of which I would like to take a few moments to express my appreciation for their help in making Bollywood Abs possible.

First of all, to Saurabuh Lubaya, whose physique you will see on the front cover, a great friend and top model. To Mahesh Rita for his amazing wealth of knowledge on Indian and Asian Bodybuilding, to the guys at my company SPN Fitness, Matt & Rebecca for their research into this project and for their proof reading skills!

Special thanks also to Abhikesh Das and to Aman Bhandari of Sykz Gym in New Delhi for allowing us to shoot at his gym.

And lastly, I'd like to thank you, the reader for the opportunity to share this book with you. I truly hope that my advice will go some way in helping you achieve your fitness goals and create that body you've always wanted. Remember, where there's a will, there's a way. You bring the will and I'll show you the way!

Yours in health,

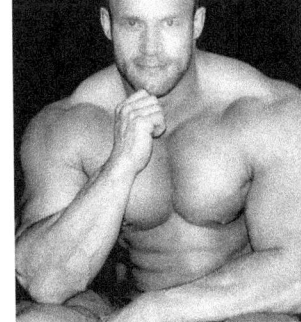

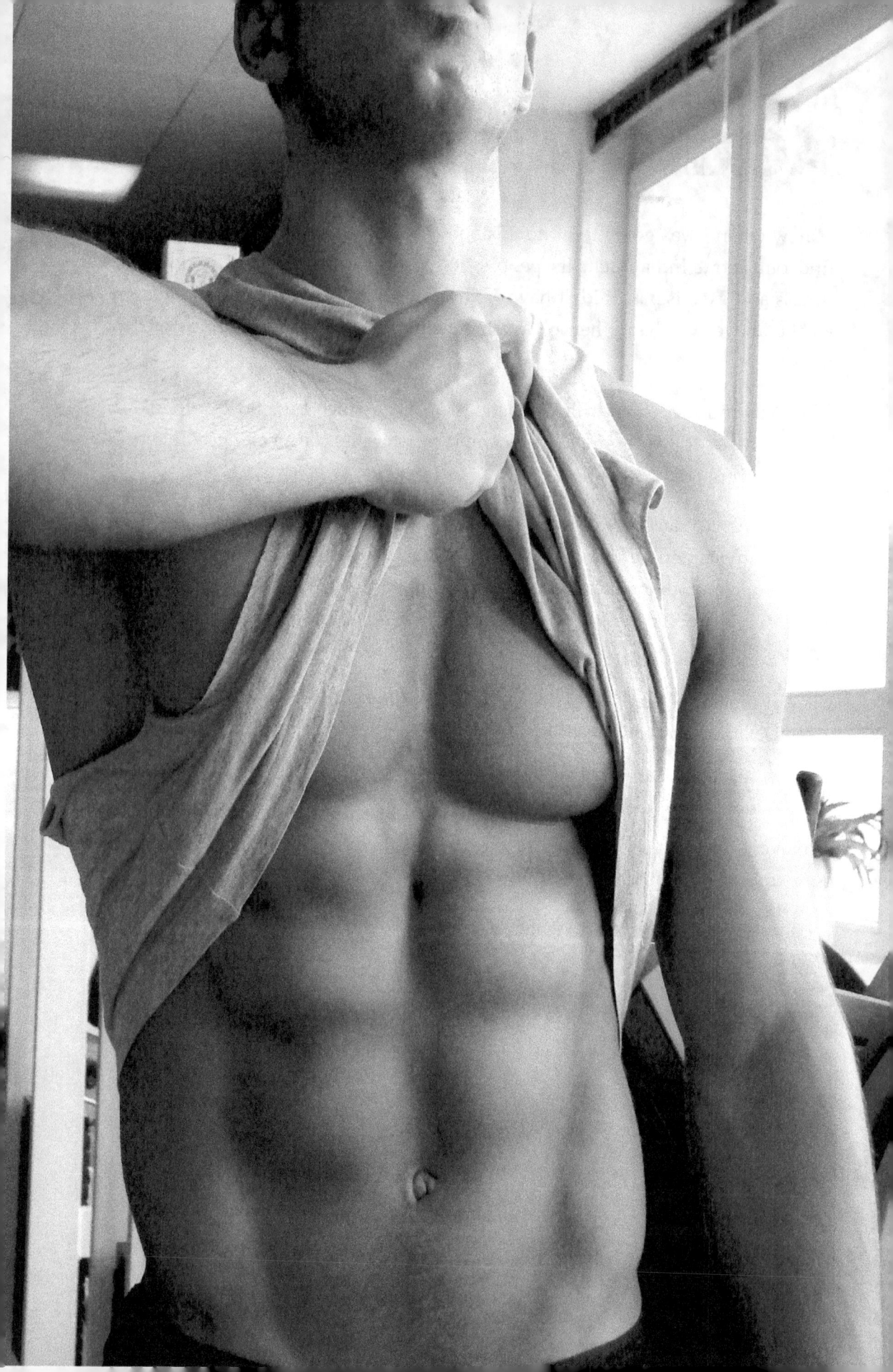

"Abs are made in the kitchen, not in the gym"

*Justin Leonard, Leonard Fitness LLC*

# INTRODUCTION

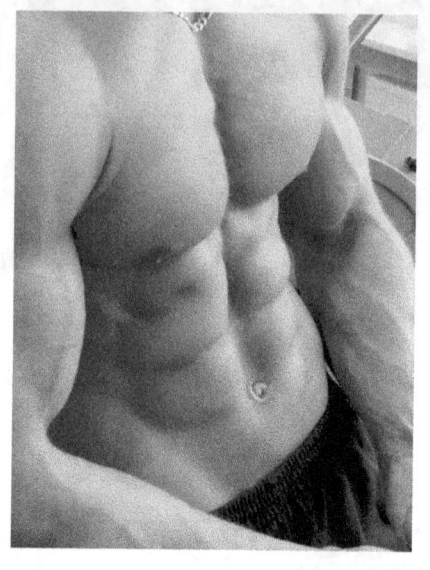

We've never met have we? Yet there is something I already know about you. I know you're serious about making a real change in your life, for the better. I know you're ready more than ever to get in the best shape you can. So let me personally welcome you to my Bollywood Abs System. As you read this book in the coming hours, days, weeks and even months, I hope to guide you to success and show you the way forward to achieve the body you desire. The journey you will take is going to be one of many exiting changes and I guarantee that if you dedicate everything into achieving this, YOU WILL finally create your BEST BODY!

I'm often asked, "Neil, how do you get great abs? What exercises will get me a six pack?" My answer now as always is very simple..."Abs are made in the kitchen, not in the gym. Forget endless ab workouts, it's your diet that will define whether you have abs or not". Before we go any further, I need you to remember this and place it in your head as I'll be coming back to it later.

In this book I am going to show you exactly how to eat and train for the ultimate physique. Never before has a book been written exclusively for the Indian market and incorporating Indian Foods! I believe this is the very reason why so many Asian men have never been able to build bigger muscles or get those rock hard abs, simply due to the fact that most magazines or books only provide a western style diet!  In this book you will be given lots of protein packed, healthy, low fat Indian Meals to help pack on the muscle....fast!

So how do you get that 'Bollywood' Body? It's a question I'm sure you've asked yourself a hundred times before but you've never actually found the answer. In all honesty there are no real secrets despite what other books or fitness magazines will have you believe. Getting in great shape comes down to having the knowledge and willpower to achieve your goal and it's in this book that I will teach and provide you with the knowledge to succeed.

There isn't a day that goes past when you're not reminded of the super slim bodies of Bollywood and Hollywood Celebrities and Sports-stars on the TV, in newspapers or in glossy magazines. Whether it's WWE Star John Cena showing his pumped body or Bollywood Legend Salman Khan flexing his pecs in the latest Bollywood Blockbuster!  It seems we are all made in some way to feel inadequate and that obtaining that very body we envy, is just another dream we will never fulfil.

Don't be fooled though, a great body is not just reserved solely for the likes of Superstars, Sports Personalities, Fitness Models or Bodybuilders, it's obtainable by everyone! And that includes YOU! What's more, you don't have to starve yourself or go on western style diet in order to achieve it. We all have the ability to change our physiques to spectacular new heights and for many of us it means only a few changes in our diet and lifestyle.

Getting abs and getting in shape takes a lot of dedication and self sacrifice, trust me, it took me sometime time to achieve it myself. It's by no means easy, especially living in a country that is still some way behind western countries when it comes to health and fitness, but it's catching up....fast! But believe me, it is obtainable by anyone who is prepared to commit time into achieving it and this is where I can help guide and mentor you into obtaining those results.

Try to view this new journey as a puzzle, where each piece fits together to create the whole picture. The pieces in this case will be each element of the program and as I guide you on the do's and dont's you will begin to collect the pieces and begin placing each one together. Whether you're looking to shape up for an upcoming special occasion or want to look and feel great for the rest of your life, *Bollywood Abs* will deliver results! Not just in the short term, but for many years to come. This is a new lifestyle and if you have the will power to make some simple changes and stick to them you will see fantastic results.

# READY TO **COMMIT?**

In a recent study of women when asked what they felt were the sexiest parts of the male body. Abs came in first (*no surprise there!*), followed by pecs, arms and bottom! There is no doubt that a set of abs really complete a physique. You can have a great chest and arms, but if your abs are lagging behind, you just won't feel or look complete. Abs not only look sexy but they complete the whole picture. So how ready are you for this *'six pack transformation'*?

You may well have already tried every abdominal exercise there is, spent many a nights crunching at the end of your bed, attempted to adopt a healthier lifestyle or diet plan, even joined a local gym in an effort to lose those excess pounds or even put some on, but it never quite happened the way you wanted it to, right? Those abs still don't show, you get discouraged and then give up!!

Don't worry, its happened to us all! But this is about to finally change. A change like you've never experienced before, a change so great that you'll be wanting to show off your new set of toned abs to everyone! And hopefully promoting my system to your friends and family!

But how ready are you? Are you fully prepared for what's ahead? As mentioned earlier, getting a great body is not easy, it takes sacrifices and here are some you need to be prepared to do:

- Change your eating habits and incorporate healthier versions of Indian Meals

- Adopt a new healthier lifestyle

- Begin a new workout/exercise regimen

- Commit and dedicate time to reaching your goal

**Are you up for it?** Great, let's begin......

There are many reasons as to why you may have purchased my book, maybe you're tired of the way you look and ready more than ever to do something about it, maybe you are totally new to a challenge like this or maybe you've reached a plateau in your workouts and just don't know which direction to head in next. Whatever the reason, you've certainly found the right program to make some very significant changes, not only in your body, but in your life too.

First off, the journey toward a fit and healthy physique must be grounded in the proper mindset. You must be **motivated**, or else you will likely give up within a matter of weeks or even days! To stay motivated, it is important to make a promise to yourself both in your mind and on paper that you will do everything in your power to live in such a way that will allow you to come closer to your goals. This means taking time to make healthier versions of your meals, working out regularly, and doing it with **confidence, conviction, and a positive attitude!!**

Whenever you start a fitness program you should always have a personal REASON to get in shape. That reason has to be clear, precise, and important enough to you to keep you motivated. If your reason isn't strong enough, your motivation will soon drop, and you will go on a downward spiral away from your goals and end up no closer to your goal than when you started!

To make real changes to your body you have to make sacrifices and these sacrifices you will be faced with daily. Whether it's making a healthier meal at home as opposed to using a street vendor, or staying at the gym those extra few minutes instead of leaving early because you want to get home to watch some TV show that you just can't afford to miss. These are sacrifices you will face and only you can be the one to make the decision. Knowing the bad habits from the good will be the factor that determines your individual success. I want you to look in the mirror in weeks from now with a smile about the reflection you see and say "I did it!" The feeling of accomplishment and the benefits of a greater body and feeling of well being are far greater than anything you could imagine. But this accomplishment will **only** come from sheer determination, commitment and sacrifice. So which is it to be? The new you? or the same you? I think I have an idea of your answer!

If you're ready, let's get to work!

# THE **BASICS**

In the Introduction I mentioned the word 'knowledge'. In order for you to have a successful journey with my system, you must make new steps each day and act on the "knowledge" that is presented in this book. Every piece of information I provide you, ultimately provides you with more 'knowledge' to succeed. The outcome of your journey is **determined by you and you only.** Laying down the

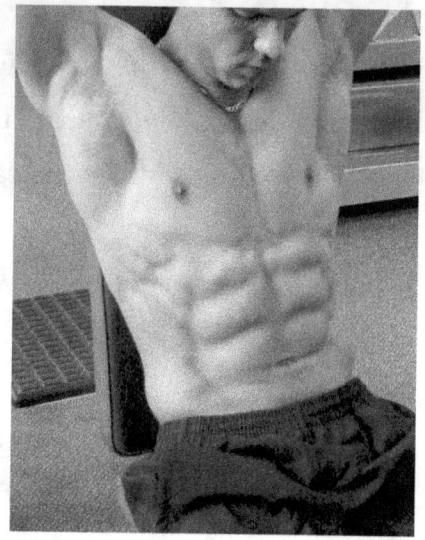

basic fundamentals of your program is essential and you must set structured goals over the course of the coming weeks, not 12 days! Don't expect to see your abs in the next five days, it won't happen. Abs are not created overnight, it takes time, so you must fully concentrate on your goals over the coming weeks.

Starting a health and fitness program is a daunting task for anyone and with so much information to digest and divulge for some it can be very overwhelming. During your quest for great abs, try not to change too much in your life too quickly. Many people, in their search for a new body make broad resolutions that require several different lifestyle changes. Quitting smoking, starting an exercise program, and dieting all in the same week can be extremely challenging and tackling any one of the above is challenging enough. If you have any of the above vices or others, you may want to try one step at a time rather than trying "cold turkey - and all at once!" Gradual change will bring about the very best results and I encourage all new trainees to consider this before jumping head first into the program.

The best way to start your journey is to take a 'before' picture of how you are now, in another week you'll take another and you'll begin a succession of progress photos to capture your progress. The changes you will see in the photos will motivate you to keep striving and pushing harder and harder.

Unfortunately many people often start their journey with precision focus and commitment, but somewhere along the way they take an alternative route and let me assure you, once you're off course, it's damn hard to get back on track! Stick to the fundamentals and the "knowledge" and you'll make the right turns.

My advice would be to begin the program by taking a week to concentrate on your Diet. This diet is going to be the most important aspect of this program and it will take time to adapt to this healthier eating. Spend the first week changing the way you cook your meals, read over the nutrition section a few times and familiarize yourself with all the listed nutrients, get into the habit of 5-6 smaller sized meals each day, drink more water and most importantly be as consistent as possible. It will take some getting used to, but for the first week it's a good idea to concentrate solely on this before implementing your training.

When week 2 arrives you'll pretty much have your diet set in stone and with a clear head you can begin your training.

## SUMMARY:

- Don't jump head first into the program, gradual changes over the coming weeks will get you on the right track.

- Take a before photo under good light. This will be the beginning of regular photos to chart your progress over the coming weeks.

- Set your goals firmly in your mind or write them down.

- Consider beginning Week one with getting used to your new diet. You can then start the training in Week 2.

# CHANGING **OLD HABITS** AND MAKING **NEW ONES!**

We all have habits in our day to day lives that we never even think twice about. We most definitely have habits when it comes to eating. And it's such habits that can make us fat or make us thin! Long term success relies heavily on eliminating bad habits and creating good ones. However, creating new habits is never easy. But let me assure you once you've put them into practice, they just get easier and easier! Opting for a lower fat chicken or vegetable curry prepared at home as opposed to a f ried Chicken dish from a street vendor or fast food restaurant will become second nature and you'll adjust just as quickly as you dropped the bad habit. To make things simple you have to provide your body with food that will nourish it and dispose of those which will contaminate it, it's that simple. When you make a change, your body reacts, it notices this and reacts with a multitude of benefits.

I must stress that this is not a 'diet', this is a new way of life, a nutritional plan you can implement for years to come, I refer to it as the *'Bollywood Abs Diet'*. Over the coming weeks you'll learn so much about how your body reacts to different foods, how they give you energy, how they make you feel tired, sluggish and irritable and how they can lift you when you're feeling low. You'll also learn about the pitfalls of foods labelled as 'low fat' or 'low calorie', such things that can make so much difference in trimming your waistline.

# FEEDING **YOUR** BODY

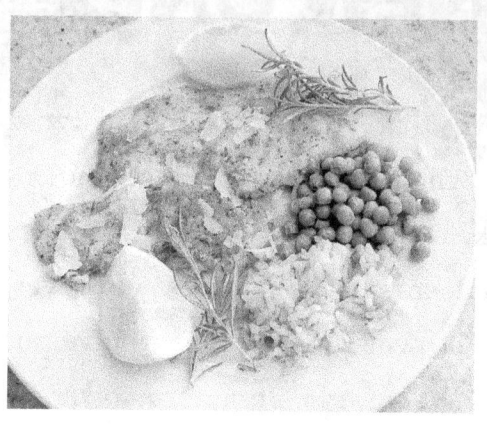

Diet accounts for as much as **80%** when getting in great shape, yes **80%**. At the beginning of this book I used a quote, can you remember what it was? In case you forgot, let me remind you. "Abs are made in the kitchen, not in the gym" YOU MUST BELIEVE THIS! IF YOU DO NOT CHANGE YOUR DIET, YOU WILL FAIL! Far too many guys simply concentrate all their efforts into training in the gym and then wonder why results just don't show. In India this is very understandable due to the tradition of very high fat foods, however, I am changing this and providing you with a simple, affordable and effective way of creating healthy Indian meals that will get you in great shape! This really is going to be the key factor that separates a great body from an average one. Knowing exactly which foods stimulate it and those that in effect destroy it, is something that I will help teach you. **The importance of correct nutrition is without doubt the core element of this program** and the more you learn about correct eating and balancing, the greater abdominal definition you will achieve. The key is basically to know which foods will feed your muscles and which will starve the fat. Good eating habits become part of a new lifestyle and it's this new lifestyle which will determine your overall success. Let's take a look at the key ingredients to form your nutrition program.

## PROTEIN

What is protein? Protein is the building block for muscle. Imagine a brick house, you can't build that house without the bricks, right? Well the same goes for your body, you can't build lean muscles without protein in sufficient quantities. Every single meal 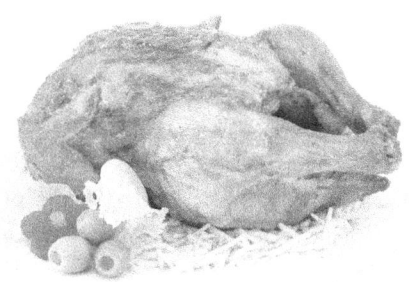 you consume from now on will contain some form of quality protein. Generally the best sources come from, chicken, turkey, fish, egg whites, soy beans and whey protein shakes and bars. For Vegetarians, Lentils, Pulses and Legumes, Veggie Burgers and Meat substitutes, Soy, Tofu, Nuts and Protein Supplements. Protein also contains essential amino acids, which work together to help you build leaner, stronger muscles. For non-meat eaters Protein Supplementation (Shakes) are strongly encouraged to help booster your protein intake enough to build muscle, I will touch more on this later.

## CARBOHYDRATES

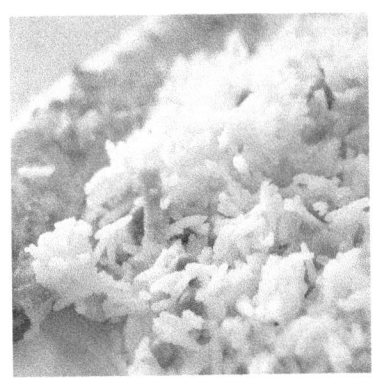 There are two types of carbohydrates, which usually causes some confusion. The first is 'Complex carbs' also known as 'slow glycemic carbs' or 'fat loss carbs.' These carbs provide the body with a constant release of energy to help you train and exercise effectively. The very best sources are rice, wholegrains, wholegrain pastas, potatoes, sweet potatoes/yams, dhal, fresh vegetables and salads. The other type are 'simple carbs', refined sugars like sodas, fruits, sweets, juices, white

flour based products like white breads, bagels, rices, naans, rotis and pastas. These carbs are converted quickly to blood sugar by your body as soon as you've digested them. These carbs provide quick energy as opposed to the 'slow carbs' which provide longer lasting energy. Usually your energy plummets rapidly with 'simple carbs'. It's these carbs that will need to be consumed at very specific times. Because of their sudden and dramatic effect, their response on the fat loss process is a negative one. When you feel the crash effects of consuming simple carbs and your energy begins to decrease this is where the problem begins to occur. You'll start to feel hungry very quickly and this is the sign that your body is calling for more blood sugar and more food. This is great if you want to put on weight and bulk up, but not if you're looking to lean out and chisel those abs!

Here's a list of good carbs and bad carbs:

## GOOD

Sweet Potato, Squash, Potato, Oatmeal, Oats, Shredded Wheat, Whole wheat Cereal, Whole wheat Pasta & Spaghetti, Brown Rice, Barley, Beans, Corn, Strawberries, Raspberries, Apples, Oranges, Melon, Avocado, Whole Wheat Bread or Pita, Cucumber, Lettuce, Celery, Cabbage, Green Peppers, Green Beans, Cauliflower, Peas, Brussels Sprouts, Spinach, Tomato, Asparagus, Broccoli, Zuccini, Onion, Watercress, Bean Sprouts, Cashews, Nuts, low fat yogurt or live yogurt

## BAD CARBS

White Flour based products, bagels, white bread, white flour chapatis and dosas, poppodums, white based pastas, snacks biscuits, sweets, desserts, fries, donuts, candy bars, chips and nachos etc.

## FAT

Fat is very much a double-edged sword meaning it can be both good for you and bad for you! Unfortunately Indian Cuisine is predominantly high in fat as most foods use large amounts of oil and and are often fried, which is not ideal for someone who wants to get in shape. Let's 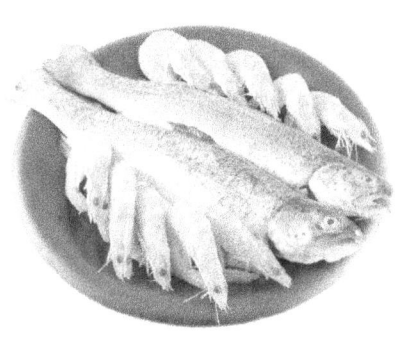 take a look at the two different types of fat. **Saturated** (Bad) and **Unsaturated**, known also as essential fatty acids (Good). Some people believe, that to live a healthy life, fat should be completely eliminated from your diet, **not true**. We actually need to feed our body with some fat to help it function properly. Let's begin with saturated fats, found all fried foods, fried breads, fast foods, fries, candy, sweets, puddings, etc. These fats are <u>not</u> required in your diet. They will do nothing but set you back and stop you from getting lean. Eating them once a week is fine, but any of the above consumed regularly will limit your progress without question. On the other hand unsaturated fats found in, all fish, nuts, seeds etc. are extremely good for you. These essential fatty acids contain omega 3 and 6 oils, which can only be consumed in food or supplements, your body cannot make these acids. And, without these omega oils your body will be unable to maximize the fat loss process. Many people when beginning a new diet often start by eating primarily low fat foods and within days they feel exhausted, irritable and even dizzy, and this is a sign that the body is craving essential fatty acids (Unsaturated fats). You may not feel like eating fish day in day out, so it's essential to purchase a good oil like, sunflower oil, cod liver, flaxseed, safflower, soy bean or canola oil. Alternatively you can purchase oils in capsules form, Cod Liver Oil Capsules is my recommended choice.

## SUGAR

**Sugar is the No.1 culprit for adding and keeping body fat!** You must make a real effort to reduce and monitor your intake of refined sugars in your diet. Where are the refined sugars? you may ask. They are everywhere! Therefore, in order to accomplish this goal we need to do the following:

- Avoid regular sodas as they contain a large amount of sugar in them. Instead, begin drinking more water (General rule of thumb 1 ounce of water per kilo of bodyweight)

- Avoid the use of table sugars, adding to tea/coffee

- Avoid eating sugary desserts or puddings

Some sugars are ok, for instance sugar from raw honey and black strap molasses because they contain certain enzymes that make them healthy. However, these sugars should still be used scarcely in your nutritional regimen. Make the commitment and limit all the sugar in your diet, there is no doubt that sugar moderation really does make the difference.

## SUGARS IN FRUIT?

The sugar found in fruit is something known as FRUCTOSE. "Fructose is broken down by the body slowly and is converted into SUCROSE and GLYCOGEN, we should not treat this type of sugar the same as table sugar, however, to get lean, you must still be careful not to eat too much fruit.

### So do I have to eliminate fruit?

Absolutely not, with fruit being such a good source of energy, fruit intake is encouraged especially on days you exercise before and after training. I will come to this a little later.

# SUMMARY:

- Correct Nutrition accounts for as much as **80%** of your success.

- PROTEIN – The Muscle Builder, eat plenty of it!

- VEGETARIAN?  Lentils, Dhal, Vegetables, Legumes, Tofu and Soy are your best sources of protein

- Using a Whey, Casein, Soy or Hemp Protein Supplement is encouraged, **these are very safe to use.**

- CARBS – Complex carbs should be used in meals, especially oats, rice cakes, vegetables, fruits.

- Simple Carbs (fruits) should only be consumed after a weight training workout to help replenish your system.

- FAT – Saturated is BAD! – Unsaturated is GOOD!

- Your last meal of the day should have no carbs.

- Cook with Extra Virgin Olive Oil, Flaxseed Oil or Canola Oil

- SUGAR – The No1 Culprit for adding body fat! Avoid eating table sugars, adding to tea, coffee, desserts or cereals. Sugars found in fruits and vegetables are fine.

- ALLOW YOURSELF ONE CHEAT DAY EACH WEEK WHERE YOU CAN ENJOY YOUR FAVORITE FOODS AND RELAX FROM THE DIET.

# BOLLYWOOD ABS DIET
## MEAL PLANNER

Ok, now here comes the part where it's time to take a look at some meal ideas for the day. You'll see both Indian and Western meals to provide variety and more options. You'll also see that five to six meals per day are required. Feel free to mix meals around to suit you, eg. Use some of the mid-afternoon meals for mid-morning or vice versa.

You will notice that each meal is given one of the following symbols:

**LOW** = LOW CARB DAY  or  **HIGH** = HIGH CARB DAY.

High Carb days require an increase in carb intake, where as, Low Carb days require less. This is called **'CARB ROTATION'** and is explained on *page 171*.

**Breakfast Meals** – *1 small glass of buttermilk can be consumed with breakfast daily*

**LOW** **Egg White Omelet** made with 8 egg whites, 2 yolks, 1 teaspoon of oil, 1 small onion chopped, 5 button mushrooms, ½ green or red pepper, white or black pepper to taste.

*Macros:  Protein: 25g  Carbs: 5g  Fat: 5g  Sodium: 0.4g*

*or*

**LOW** **Indian Style Microwave Omelet** made with 8 egg whites, 2 yolks, 1 teaspoon of oil, 1 small onion chopped, 2 green chillies finely chopped, few sprigs of fresh coriander, 1 tablespoon of milk, pepper to taste, 1 tablespoon of butter or low fat spread

*or*

**HIGH** **Breakfast Chapati** - Whole-wheat chapatis x 2 with four scrambled egg whites. Tablespoon of Salsa, low fat shredded cheese and low fat sour cream. Plus Protein shake, 1 scoop in water

*Macros:  Protein: 25-35g   Carbs: 30g   Fat: 4g   Sodium: 1g*

*or*

**HIGH** **Wholewheat or Wholegrain Cereal** (80g) with 200ml of skimmed or Skimmed milk, plus 2 scoops of Whey Protein powder in a shake. Tea/Coffee (no sugar added)

*Macros:  Protein: 25-35g   Carbs: 35g   Fat: 2g   Sodium: 0.4g*

*or*

**HIGH** **Western Style Egg White Omelet** made with 6 egg whites and 1 yolk. Add grated ham, onion, spinach or diced chicken and pepper. 1/2 slices of whole-wheat toast.

*Macros:  Protein: 25g   Carbs: 30g   Fat: 4g   Sodium: 0.8g*

*or*

**HIGH** **Oats** - 80g of Instant Oatmeal/Oats (Unsweetened and Unflavored) with protein shake (2 scoops in water).

*Macros:  Protein: 25-35g   Carbs: 40g   Fat: 2g   Sodium: 0.4g*

*or*

**HIGH** **Whey Shake** (2 scoops of protein powder 60g) with piece of fruit (apple, banana, muskmelon, apricots, peach, mango, pear, avocado or orange) (Peanut Butter may be added to your shake)

*Macros:  Protein: 40g   Carbs: 40g   Fat: 7g of which 5g is good fats   Sodium: 0.6g*

*or*

**HIGH** **Chapati Burger** – 2 slices of lean bacon, 2 x 8 inch wholewheat chapatis. One-two scoop of Whey Powder in a separate shake (150ml water). Note, bacon can be replaced with any other type of lean meat.

*Macros:  Protein: 25-35g   Carbs: 35g   Fat: 2g   Sodium: 1g*

*or*

**LOW** **Wholegrain Bagel** with 1 teaspoon of Crunchy Peanut Butter. Protein Shake with 2 scoops of whey powder and 200 ml of water.

*Macros:  Protein: 25-35g   Carbs: 40g   Fat: 2g   Sodium: 0.5g*

## Mid Morning Meals

**LOW** **Chicken Chapati** - 100g of Turkey or Chicken in 1 x Wholewheat Chapati (8 inch) with lettuce or salad + 1 x scoop of Whey Powder in a Shake

*Macros: Protein: 40g Carbs: 11g Fat: 1.5g Sodium: 1.0g*

*or*

**HIGH** **Maida & Urad Dosa with Chicken or Tuna** - 1/2 cup of Split black gram (Urad Dal), 1 cup of wholegrain flour, pinch or two of salt, 2 teaspoon of oil - 1/2 tsp per dosa or use Pam Spray if available or grape seed oil spray. Add 120g of Chicken or tuna fish

*Macros: Protein: 30g Carbs: 38g Fat: 8.9g Sodium: 1.5g* **(Based on 2 Dosas)**

*or*

**LOW** **Tuna Salad** – 115g Tin of water packed Tuna fish mixed with half a spoon of low fat mayonnaise, with freshly squeezed lemon juice with diced salad or 2 x wholewheat chapatis

*Macros: Protein: 25-35g Carbs: 25g Fat: 4g Sodium: 0.9g*

*or*

**LOW** **Whey Shake with handful of nuts** or sunflower/pumpkin seeds

*Macros: Protein: 40g Carbs: 10g Fat: 6g of which 5g is good fats Sodium: 0.4g*

*or*

**HIGH** **Cottage Cheese Snack** - 200g of low fat cottage cheese with raw carrot and celery sticks or 4-5 Rice Cakes or idlis or dosas

*Macros: Protein: 25g Carbs: 25g Fat: 4g Sodium: 1g*

*or*

**HIGH** **Whey Protein Shake** with 200 ml of cold water sand 2-3 heaped tablespoons of oats

*Macros: Protein: 25-35g Carbs: 30g Fat: 2g Sodium: 0.4g*

*or*

**HIGH** **Keema Curry Lentil Soup** - 10 oz. ground turkey or chicken (275g), 1 small onion chopped, ½ teaspoon of curry powder, 2 cloves garlic, ½ teaspoon of cumin, ¼ teaspoon ginger, pinch of cinnamon, pinch of cloves, pinch of cayenne pepper, Salt and pepper to taste, 1 carrot shredded, 2 celery sticks, 1/2 cup of dried lentils, 2 medium potatoes chopped, 4 tablespoons of tomato sauce, 2 cups of chicken broth

*Macros Per Portion (Makes 4 portions): Protein: 23g  Carbs: 34g  Fat: 2g  Sodium: 0.7g*

*or*

**HIGH** **Chicken Burrito** - Whole-wheat tortilla with 100g sliced, cooked chicken or turkey breast. Tablespoon of Salsa.

*Macros:  Protein: 25-30g  Carbs: 25g  Fat: 3.5g  Sodium: 0.7g*

*or*

**HIGH** **Lean Meat Roll or Sandwich** with 75-125g of Tuna, Chicken, lean ham or Turkey + Protein Shake

*Macros:  Protein: 15-30g  Carbs: 25g  Fat: 4g  Sodium: 0.8g*

## Lunch Meals:

**HIGH** **Tandoori Chicken** - 200g of boneless chicken breast, skinned and cut into sizeable chunks, ¼ tsp garam masala,  ¼ tsp of ginger pulp, ¼ tsp of garlic pulp, ¼ tsp of chili powder, pinch of turmeric, pinch of salt, 50ml of low fat yogurt, ¼ tablespoon of lemon juice, chopped fresh coriander, ¼ tab of oil. Served with Pea and Mushroom Pilau Rice

*Macros:  Protein: 35g  Carbs: 45g  Fat: 9g  Sodium: 1.6g*

*or*

**LOW** **Prawns with Vegetables** - 8 King Prawns Peeled, ½ tablespoon chopped fresh coriander, 1 Green chili, 1 tablespoon of lemon juice, ¾ tablespoon of oil, 1 medium courgette sliced, 1 medium onion cut into chunks, some cherry tomatoes, 3 baby corn on the cobs. To make as a High Carb Meal simply add a rice or lentil side

*Macros:  Protein: 25g  Carbs: 5g  Fat: 7g  Sodium: 1.6g*

*or*

**LOW** **Pineapple Chicken Kebabs** - 200g of boneless chicken skinned and cubed, 60g of canned pineapple, ¼ tsp ground cumin, ¼ tsp ground coriander, ¼ tsp chili powder, ¼ tsp garlic pulp, ¼ tsp salt, ½ tablespoon natural low fat yogurt, ½ tablespoon of chopped fresh coriander, ¼ of yellow or green pepper seeded, ½ an onion, 2 cherry tomatoes, ¼ tablespoon of oil. To make as a High Carb Meal simply add a rice or lentil side

*Macros: Protein: 30g  Carbs: 15g  Fat: 6.5g   Sodium: 1.0g*

*or*

**LOW** **Karahi Chicken with Mint** - 200g of chicken breast, skinned and cut into strips, 75ml of water, ½ tablespoon of oil, 2 spring onions chopped, ¼ tsp of shredded root ginger, ¼ tsp of crushed dried chillies, ¾ tablespoon of lemon juice, ¼ tablespoon chopped fresh coriander, ¼ tablespoon choped fresh mint, 1 tomato skinned, seeded and roughly chopped, pinch of salt, mint, coriander to garnish. To make as a High Carb Meal simply add a rice or lentil side.

*Macros: Protein: 30g  Carbs: 5g  Fat: 8g   Sodium: 1.1g*

*or*

**HIGH** **Chicken/Turkey with Rice** - 150g of Chicken or Turkey Breast with either Brown Rice/Wholewheat spaghetti or Pasta with Vegetables. Lemon Juice or Low-Fat Sauce

*Macros: Protein: 30g  Carbs: 45g  Fat: 5g   Sodium: 1.6g*

*or*

**LOW** **Tuna Salad** - 150g Tin of water packed tuna mixed with teaspoon of fat free mayo or salad cream with lettuce, cucumber and tomato. Relish may be added.

*Macros: Protein: 30g  Carbs: 15g  Fat: 3g   Sodium: 0.9g*

*or*

**HIGH** **Whey Protein Shake** (2 scoops 60g)) with 200 ml of cold water or skimmed milk + 1 piece of fruit: Apple, Pear, Orange or Peach

*Macros: Protein: 40g  Carbs: 30g  Fat: 3g   Sodium: 0.5g*

*or*

**LOW** **Sandwich** - 2 slices of Wholewheat Bread with either 100g of steak, turkey or tuna fish and salad. Protein Shake

*Macros: Protein: 25g  Carbs: 35g  Fat: 5g   Sodium: 1g*

*or*

**LOW** **Fruit Salad** - Mixed fruit in a small bowl with 2 x scoops of Whey Protein in a shake

*Macros: Protein: 30g  Carbs: 30g  Fat: 2.4g   Sodium: 0.7g*

*or*

**LOW** **Chicken/Turkey in Wholewheat Tortilla** 100-125g of sliced, cooked chicken or turkey breast. Tablespoon of Salsa.

*Macros:  Protein: 30-35g  Carbs: 15g  Fat: 3g    Sodium: 0.8g*

*or*

**HIGH** **White Fish with Potato** – 150g of white fish served with baked or sweet potato and small serving of salad or vegetables. Squeeze of lemon juice to flavor.

*Macros:  Protein: 40g  Carbs: 40g  Fat: 7g    Sodium: 1.0g*

## Mid Afternoon Meals:

**LOW** **Tuna Salad** - Half a tin of water packed tuna fish (70g) with raw vegetables or loose leaf lettuce/cucumber/tomato or celery.

*Macros:  Protein: 20g  Carbs: 15g  Fat: 2g    Sodium: 0.8g*

*or*

**LOW** **Protein Shake** - 1 scoop of Whey Protein added to 200-300 ml of cold water or skimmed milk + handful of mixed nuts and raspberries or strawberries.

*Macros:  Protein: 20g  Carbs: 20g  Fat: 7g    Sodium: 0.7g*

*or*

**HIGH** **Chicken Wholemeal Chapatis** - 125-150g of Chicken/Turkey with 2 x Wholemeal Chapatis x 2. Tablespoon of Salsa.

*Macros:  Protein: 30-35g  Carbs: 30g  Fat: 3g    Sodium: 0.8g*

*or*

**HIGH** **Baked Potato with Spicy Cottage Cheese** - 1 medium baking potato, 75g of low fat cottage cheese, ½ teaspoon of tomato puree, pinch of ground cumin, pinch of ground coriander, pinch of chili powder, touch of oil, pinch of onion and mustard seeds, 1 curry leaf, 10ml of water

*Macros:  Protein: 12g  Carbs: 25g  Fat: 5g    Sodium: 1.2g*

*or*

**LOW** **Cottage Cheese** - 4 x Rice Cakes with 150g of low fat cottage or with 2 x Wholewheat chapatis

*With Rice Cakes:  Macros:  Protein: 20g  Carbs: 20g  Fat: 2.5g  Sodium: 1.0g*

*With chapatis  Macros:  Protein: 20g  Carbs: 35g  Fat: 6.5g  Sodium: 1.4g*

## Dinner Meals: *You can add any rice/side to all low carb meals to increase carbs for high days*

**LOW** **Tandoori Chicken Kebabs** - 200g of chicken breast, skinned and cubed, ¼ tablespoon of lemon juice, 1 tablespoon of tandoori paste, 1 tablespoon of low fat yogurt, ¼ garlic clove crushed, ½ tablespoon of freshly chopped coriander, pinch of salt and black pepper, ½ an onion cut into wedges and separated into layers, a little oil brushed, fresh coriander sprigs to garnish.

*Macros:  Protein: 25-30g  Carbs: 4g  Fat: 8.0g  Sodium: 1.2g*

*or*

**LOW** **Chicken Balti with Spicy Lentil Sauce** - 200g of chicken breast, skinned and cubed, ½ tablespoon of chana dhal, 15g or 1oz of masoor dhal, ¼ tablespoon of oil, 1 medium onion chopped, ¼ tsp garlic pulp, ¼ tsp ginger pulp, pinch of ground turmeric, ½ tsp of chili powder, ¼ tsp of garam masala, pinch of ground coriander, pinch of salt, 1 tablespoon of fresh coriander leaves, ½ green chili, seeded and chopped, 1 tablespoon of lemon juice, 75ml of water, 1 tomato peeled and halved

*Macros:  Protein: 25-30g  Carbs: 20g  Fat: 7.5g  Sodium: 1.1g*

*or*

**LOW** **King Prawn Bhoona** - 5-6 king prawns thawed and peeled or 125-150g of peeled prawns, ¼ tsp paprika, ¼ tsp ginger pulp, pinch of salt, 1 tablespoon of natural low fat yogurt, ¼ tablespoon of oil, 1 medium onion sliced, pinch of fennel seeds crushed, ¼ piece of cinnamon bark (optional), ¼ tsp garlic pulp, ¼ tsp chili powder, 1/3 a yellow or red pepper seeded and roughly chopped, fresh coriander leaves to garnish. *Serve with Rice Dish or side to increase to high carb meal.*

*Macros:  Protein: 25-30g  Carbs: 15g  Fat: 4.0g  Sodium: 1.2g*

*or*

**LOW** **Monkfish with Vegetables** - 150g of Monkfish, ½ tablespoon of oil, ½ medium onion sliced, ¼ tsp garlic pulp, ¼ tsp ground cumin, ¼ tsp ground coriander, ¼ tsp chili powder, ½ tablespoon of fresh fenugreek leaves, 1 tomato seeded and sliced, ½ a courgette sliced, pinch of salt, ¼ tablespoon of lime juice

*Macros:  Protein: 25-30g  Carbs: 8.0g   Fat: 3.0g    Sodium: 0.8g*

*or*

**LOW** **Fish and Vegetable Kebabs** - 150g of white fish fillets like cod or haddock, 1 tablespoon of lemon juice, ¼ tsp of ginger pulp, ½ green chili very finely chopped, ¼ tablespoon of very finely chopped fresh coriander, ¼ tablespoon of very finely chopped fresh mint, ¼ tsp of ground coriander, pinch of salt, 1/3 a red or green pepper, ¼ of a medium cauliflower, 3 button mushrooms, 2 cherry tomatoes or half a medium tomato, ¼ tablespoon of oil, ¼ of a lime used to garnish

*Macros:  Protein: 25-30g  Carbs: 8.0g   Fat: 4.0g    Sodium: 0.8g*

*or*

**LOW** **Tuna Curry** - 125-150g can of tinned tuna in brine drained, ¼ of an onion, ½ a red or green pepper, ½ tablespoon oil, pinch of cumin seeds, pinch of ground cumin, pinch of ground coriander, pinch of chili powder, pinch of salt, ½ a garlic clove crushed, ¼ green chili finely chopped, ¼ inch of root ginger grated, pinch of garam masala, ¼ of lemon juice, ½ tablespoon of chopped fresh coriander, plus a little to garnish, Pitta breads with Raita to serve

*Macros:  Protein: 30g  Carbs: 4g   Fat: 6.5g    Sodium: 1.2g*

*or*

**HIGH** **Lean Wholewheat Chapatis** – 100-125g of Extra Lean Minced Beef or Turkey with chopped onion, finely chopped garlic, chili powder, kidney beans, chili peppers. 3-4 Whole-wheat Chapatis. Lettuce, grated low fat cheese and sliced tomatoes.

*Macros:  Protein: 25-30g  Carbs: 35g   Fat: 2.5g    Sodium: 1.0g*

*or*

**HIGH** **Masala Steak** – 250g of boneless Mutton or Beef from the Round portion cut into steaks, 1 medium size onion sliced, 1 cup of water, Salt to taste, 1 tbsp Oil, ¼ teaspoon ginger paste, ¼ teaspoon garlic paste, ½ teaspoon coriander powder, ¼ teaspoon cumin powder, ¼ teaspoon turmeric powder, pepper to taste. 1 large baked potato. Peas or corn can be added.

*Macros:  Protein: 30g  Carbs: 35g   Fat: 9.0g    Sodium: 1.6g*

*or*

**HIGH** **Western Style Steak** - 200g Beef Undercut or Sirloin steak, ¼ teaspoon turmeric powder, 1 teaspoon fresh pepper, 1 tablespoon oil, 1 small onion sliced finely, 1 small tomatoes chopped, 1 large baked potato. Peas or corn can be added.

*Macros:  Protein: 30g  Carbs: 35g   Fat: 9.0g     Sodium: 1.6g*

*or*

**LOW** **Tuna Burgers** - 130g of tin of water packed tuna drained, 1 egg white, 1 Tbs low fat pancake mix, salt free seasoning, pepper mixed together formed into a patty and cooked in frying pan with low fat spray served with vegetables.

*Macros:  Protein: 25g  Carbs: 25g   Fat: 2.5g     Sodium: 1.0g*

*or*

**LOW** **Chicken Breast & Potato** - 125g of Skinless Chicken Breast served with baked or Sweet Potato and mixed vegetables. You may have Sweet Potato fries, cut in chunks and grill.

*Macros:  Protein: 30g  Carbs: 25g   Fat: 1.5g     Sodium: 1.0g*

*or*

**HIGH** **Minced Mutton and Rice** - 100-125g of Lean Ground Mutton/Beef mixed with baby tomatoes and basil with 100g of brown basmati rice and 50g of mixed vegetables stir fried

*Macros:  Protein: 25g  Carbs: 40g   Fat: 2.5g     Sodium: 1.0g*

*or*

**HIGH** **Western Fish with Potato & Vegetables** - 125-150g of Grilled or Baked Trout, Salmon, Haddock or Cod served with lemon juice, baked potato and vegetables. Lemon juiced can be used for taste.

*Macros:  Protein: 35-40g  Carbs: 35-40g   Fat: 7g     Sodium: 1.2g*

*or*

**HIGH** **125-150g of Sirloin, Fillet or Rump Steak** served with vegetables or salad (oven baked fries once weekly) Steak can be peppered or seasoned to your choice

*Macros:  Protein: 30-40g  Carbs: 25g   Fat: 5g     Sodium: 1.0g*

*or*

**`HIGH`** **Mild Chicken Curry** – 125g of Diced chicken breast with curry powder, finely chopped onions, fat-free natural yogurt (2 tablespoons), paprika, and brown basmati rice (80g).

*Macros:  Protein: 30g  Carbs: 40g  Fat: 5.0g    Sodium: 1.4g*

*or*

**`LOW`** **Steak Chapati** - 125g of Steak served in 1 x Wholewheat Chapati (8 inch) served with salad and low fat relish

*Macros:  Protein: 30g  Carbs: 12g  Fat: 6g    Sodium: 1.0g*

## Supper Meals (Optional) This meal must be low carbohydrate

**`H-L`** **Protein Shake** - 2 scoops of Protein powder (60g) added to 200-300 ml of cold water or skimmed Milk

*Macros:  Protein: 40g  Carbs: 5g  Fat: 2.0g    Sodium: 0.4g*

*or*

**`H-L`** **Rice Cakes or Wholewheat Chapati** with 150-200g of low fat cottage cheese. *Macros:  Protein: 20-25g  Carbs: 15g  Fat: 2.0g    Sodium: 1.0g*

*or*

**`H-L`** **Tuna Salad** - Half a tin (70g) of water packed tuna mixed with lettuce, cucumber or mixed green salad. Olive oil can be added.

*Macros:  Protein: 17g  Carbs: 5-10g  Fat: 2.0g    Sodium: 0.7g*

*or*

**`H-L`** **Low Fat Cottage cheese** (200g) with Raspberries or gooseberries

*Macros:  Protein: 25g  Carbs: 7g  Fat: 2.0g    Sodium: 1.0g*

*or*

**`H-L`** **Egg White Omelet** made with 5 egg whites, pepper, spinach and diced tomato (To increase the protein content add more egg whites. The white from a small egg = 4g of protein)

*Macros:  Protein: 20g  Carbs: 10g  Fat: 2.0g    Sodium: 0.7g*

# VEGETARIAN
## MEAL PLANNER

You will notice that each meal is given one of the following symbols:

**LOW** = LOW CARB DAY or **HIGH** = HIGH CARB DAY.

High Carb days require an increase in carb intake, whereas, Low Carb days require less. This is called **'CARB ROTATION'** and is explained on *page 171*.

**Breakfast Meals** – *1 small glass of buttermilk can be consumed with breakfast daily*

**LOW** **Upma Style Oats** - Steel Cut Oats 40g or half a cup, Clarified butter/Ghee ½ tbsp, Yellow Mustard seed ½ tbsp, ½ tsp Split Black Gram (Urad Dal), ½ tsp Hot Chili Peppers chopped finely, 2 slices of Ginger Root shredded, Pinch of salt, pinch of Sugar, 5 fresh curry leaves cut in half, 1 tsp of shredded coconut for garnish.

*Macros: Protein: 34g  Carbs: 7.5g  Fat: 7.2g  Sodium: 0.4g*

*or*

**HIGH** **Upma** - Olive Oil, 1 tbsp or Ghee, 1 tsp Yellow Mustard seed, 1 tsp Split black gram (Urad dal), 1 red ot chili cut in half, Fresh green chili Peppers, 1 pepper split in half, 1 cup of Cream of Wheat Cereal (Farina, Soji), 1 cup of hot water (8 fl oz), pinch of salt, 2 teaspoon of ginger root (optional). Fresh curry leaf, 5 leaves ripped in halves.

*Macros: Protein: 4g  Carbs: 25g  Fat: 5g  Sodium: 1.8g*

*or*

**HIGH** **Scrambled Tofu Burrito/Chapati** - ½ yellow onion, diced, ½ green bell pepper diced, 1 block tofu drained and pressed, 2 tbsp oil or margarine, 1 tsp garlic powder, 1 tsp onion powder, 1 tbsp light soy sauce, 2 tbsp nutritional yeast, ½ tsp turmeric (optional). Served with either Wholewheat Burrito or Chapati

*Macros:  Protein: 25g   Carbs: 30g   **Fat: 24g of which 21.5g is good fats**    Sodium: 1.5g*

*or*

**LOW** **Spinach & Lentil Soup** - Olive Oil ½ tbsp, Garlic 1 clove chopped finely, ½ an onion chopped, Pepper powder, paprika and cayenne - pinch of all, Coriander powder ½ tsp, Split red Lentils ½ cup, Red Ripe Tomatoes ½  cup - chopped or sliced, Frozen Spinach 5oz, Ginger Root ½ tsp grated, Cilantro 1 tbsp

*Macros:  Protein: 6g   Carbs: 16g   Fat: 3.2g    Sodium: 1g*

*or*

**HIGH** **Wholewheat or Wholegrain Cereal** (80g) with 200ml of Soy Milk or similar, plus 2 scoops of Whey , Soy or Hemp Protein powder in a shake. Tea/Coffee (no sugar added)

*Macros:  Protein: 25-35g   Carbs: 35g   Fat: 2g    Sodium: 0.4*

*or*

**HIGH** **Oats** - 80g of Instant Oatmeal/Oats (Unsweetened and Unflavored) in Soy Milk or similar with protein shake (2 scoops in water).

*Macros:  Protein: 25-35g   Carbs: 40g   Fat: 2g    Sodium: 0.4g*

*or*

**HIGH** **Whey Shake** (2 scoops of protein powder 60g) with piece of fruit (apple, banana, muskmelon, apricots, peach, mango, pear, avocado or orange) (Peanut Butter may be added to your shake)

*Macros:  Protein: 40g   Carbs: 40g   Fat: 7g of which 5g is good fats    Sodium: 0.6g*

*or*

**LOW** **Mattar Panir with Chives**– 4 oz of frozen peas, 2 oz of fresh panir, 1 teaspoon of olive oil, 1 small onion chopped, ¼ ginger root peeled and shredded, Pinch of cumin powder or seeds, Pinch of coriander powder or seeds, Pinch of cayenne pepper, ¼ sprig of fresh cilantro, Pinch of turmeric, 2 tbsp of Philadelphia Chives and Onion Cream Cheese,  1 small tomato sliced, diced and crushed

*Macros:  Protein: 9.0g   Carbs: 11g   Fat: 7.3g    Sodium: 1.8g*

*or*

**HIGH** **Wholegrain Bagel** with 1 teaspoon of Crunchy Peanut Butter.

Protein Shake with 2 scoops of whey powder and 200 ml of water.

*Macros:  Protein: 25-35g  Carbs: 40g  Fat: 2g  Sodium: 0.5g*

## Mid Morning Meals

**HIGH** **Maida & Urad Dosa with Tofu** - ½ cup of Split black gram (Urad Dal), 1 cup of wholegrain flour, pinch or two of salt, 2 teaspoon of oil - ½ tsp per dosa or use Pam Spray if available or grape seed oil spray. Add 120g of tofu to your dosa/s

*Macros:  Protein: 21g  Carbs: 38g  Fat: 8.9g  Sodium: 1.2g  (Based on 2 Dosas)*

*or*

**HIGH** **Red Lentil Dhal with Wholemeal Chapati** - 3 tablespoons peanut oil, 1 medium yellow onion, 1 tablespoon fresh ginger grated, 4 garlic cloves minced, pinch of salt, 1 cup dried red lentils, 2 tablespoon tomato paste, 4-5 cups veg broth, 5 plum tomatoes chopped, Juice of 1 lime, 1 cup lightly packed chopped fresh cilantro.  (See Wholemeal chapati Recipe in Side Dishes Section)

*Macros:  Protein: 14g  Carbs: 36g  Fat: 4g  Sodium: 0.8g*

*or*

**LOW** **Tofu & Vegetable Stir Fry with Ginger** - ¾ cup soy sauce, ½ cup lemon juice, 1 tbsp fresh ginger, grated or minced, 1 block firm or extra-firm tofu well pressed and cut into 1 inch cubes, 2 tbsp vegetable or olive oil, 1/2 cauliflower, chopped, 1 bunch broccoli chopped, 2 carrots sliced, 1 onion, chopped, 1 bell pepper sliced, 1 cup snow peas, 1 cup mushrooms sliced, 3 green onions (scallions) sliced. *(Rice can be added to this dish, allow 30g of extra carbs)*

*Macros:  Protein: 25g  Carbs: 20g  Fat: 24.5g of which 21.0g is good fats  Sodium: 1.5g*

*or*

**LOW** **Whey, Soy or Hemp Protein Shake with handful of nuts** or sunflower/pumpkin seeds.

*Macros:  Protein: 25-35g  Carbs: 10g  Fat: 6g of which 5g is good fats  Sodium: 0.4g*

*or*

**HIGH** **Cottage Cheese Snack -** 200g of low fat cottage cheese with raw carrot and celery sticks or 4-5 Rice Cakes or idlis or dosas

*Macros: Protein: 25g  Carbs: 25g  Fat: 4g  Sodium: 1g*

*or*

**HIGH** **Whey, Soy or Hemp Protein Shake** (2 scoops 60g) with 200 ml of cold water sand 2-3 heaped tablespoons of oats

*Macros: Protein: 40g  Carbs: 35g  Fat: 2g  Sodium: 0.4g*

*or*

**HIGH** **Fruit & Yogurt Mix -** Mixed bowl of fruit, gooseberry, mango, raspberries, muskmelon (galia) or watermelon with 75g of low fat natural yogurt.

*Macros: Protein: 16g  Carbs: 35g  Fat: 3g  Sodium: 0.7g*


## Lunch Meals:

**LOW** **Sweet & Sour Vegetables & Tofu Kebabs -** ½ Green Pepper seeded and cut into squares, 4 cherry tomatoes, 4 cauliflower florets, 4 cubes of tofu or panir, 4 pineapple chunks.

*Macros: Protein: 8g  Carbs: 11g  Fat: 4g  Sodium: 1.2g*

*or*

**HIGH** **Baked Potato with Spicy Cottage Cheese -** 1 medium baking potato, 75g of low fat cottage cheese, ½ teaspoon of tomato puree, pinch of ground cumin, pinch of ground coriander, pinch of chili powder, touch of oil, pinch of onion and mustard seeds, 1 curry leaf, 10ml of water.

*Macros: Protein: 12g  Carbs: 25g  Fat: 4.8g  Sodium: 1.4g*

*or*

**HIGH** **Kidney Bean Curry -** 60g tinned red kidney beans, ½ tablespoon of oil, pinch of cumin seeds, ¼ onion thinly sliced, ½ green chili finely chopped, ½ a garlic clove crushed, ½ tablespoon of curry paste, pinch of ground cumin, pinch of ground coriander, pinch of chili powder, pinch of salt, 100g of chopped tomatoes, fresh coriander to garnish.

*Macros: Protein: 18g  Carbs: 35g  Fat: 8.0g  Sodium: 1.0g*

*or*

**LOW** Spinach Dhal - 45g of yellow split peas, 45ml of water, touch of oil, pinch of black mustard seeds, ½ an onion thinly sliced, ½ garlic clove crushed, ¼ inch piece of root ginger grated or pinch of ground ginger, ¼ red chili finely chopped, 80g of canned or frozen spinach, pinch of chili powder, pinch of ground coriander, pinch of garam masala, pinch of salt.

*Macros: Protein: 8g Carbs: 20g Fat: 2.5g Sodium: 1.1g*

*or*

**HIGH** Balti Potatoes with Aubergines - 4-5 Baby Potatoes, 1-2 Small Aubergines, ¼ red pepper, touch of oil, ½ mediun onion sliced, 1-2 curry leaves, pinch of onion seeds, pinch of crushed coriander seeds, pinch of cumin seeds, ¼ teaspoon of ginger pulp, ¼ teaspoon of garlic pulp, pinch of crushed dried red chillies, ¼ tablespoon chopped fresh fenugreek, pinch of chopped fresh coriander, ¼ tablespoon natural low fat yogurt, fresh coriander leaves to garnish.

*Macros: Protein: 8g Carbs: 35g Fat: 4.7g Sodium: 1.1g*

*or*

**LOW** Stir Fry with Cauliflower & Carrot - 1 medium carrot, ¼ small cauliflower cut into florets, touch of oil, ¼ small cinnamon stick, ½ cardamom pod, touch of black pepper, pinch of salt, 1oz or 25g of peas, ¼ tablespoon of lemon juice, pinch of fresh coriander and some to garnish.

*Macros: Protein: 8g Carbs: 10g Fat: 4.2g Sodium: 0.9g*

*or*

**LOW** Vegetables, Beans & Curry Leaves - Touch of oil, 1-2 curry leaves, 1 garlic clove sliced, 1 dried red chili, pinch of onion seeds, pinch of fenugreek seeds, 1 fresh green chili chopped, 40g or 1oz of canned red kidney beans, ½ medium carrot cut into strips, 1 green bean sliced, ½ medium red pepper seeded and cut into strips, pinch of salt, squeeze of lemon juice.

*Macros: Protein: 8g Carbs: 15g Fat: 3.6g Sodium: 1.0g*

# Mid Afternoon Meals:

**LOW** **Whey, Soy or Hemp Protein Shake** - 1 scoop of Protein added to 200-300 ml of cold water or skimmed milk + handful of mixed nuts and raspberries/strawberries.

*Macros:  Protein: 20g  Carbs: 20g  Fat: 7g   Sodium: 0.7g*

*or*

**HIGH** **Red Lentil Dhal with Wholemeal Chapati** - 3 tablespoons peanut oil, 1 medium yellow onion, 1 tablespoon fresh ginger grated, 4 garlic cloves minced, 1 teaspoon salt, 1 cup dried red lentils, 2 tablespoon tomato paste, 4-5 cups veg broth, 5 plum tomatoes chopped, Juice of 1 lime, 1 cup lightly packed chopped fresh cilantro.  (See Wholemeal Chapati Recipe in Side Dishes Section)

*Macros:  Protein: 14g  Carbs: 36g  Fat: 4g   Sodium: 0.8g*

*or*

**HIGH** **Baked Potato with Spicy Cottage Cheese**  - 1 medium baking potato, 75g of low fat cottage cheese, ½ teaspoon of tomato puree, pinch of ground cumin, pinch of ground coriander, pinch of chili powder, touch of oil, pinch of onion and mustard seeds, 1 curry leaf, 10ml of water

*Macros:  Protein: 12g  Carbs: 25g  Fat: 5g   Sodium: 1.2g*

*or*

**LOW** **Cottage Cheese** - 4 x Rice Cakes with 150g of low fat cottage

*Macros:  Protein: 20g  Carbs: 20g  Fat: 2.5g   Sodium: 1.0g*

# Dinner Meals: *You can add any rice/side to all low carb meals to increase carbs for high days*

**LOW** **Low Fat Vegetable Curry** - ½ teaspoon of oil, pinch of mustard and cumin seeds, ½ an onion thinly sliced, ½ curry leaf, ½ chopped green chili, ¼ piece of root ginger finely chopped, ¼ tablespoon of curry paste, ½ small cauliflower cut into small florets, ½ a carrot thinly sliced, 30g of french beans sliced, pinch of ground turmeric, pinch of chili powder, pinch of salt, ½ a tomato finely chopped, handful of thawed frozen peas, 40ml of vegetable stock.

*Macros:  Protein: 8g   Carbs: 12g   Fat: 5.5g   Sodium: 1.2g*

*or*

**HIGH** **Vegetable Kashmiri** - ½ teaspoon of cumin seeds, 2 black peppercorns, ½ green cardamon pod (seeds only), ½ inch cinnamon stick, pinch of grated nutmeg, ½ tablespoon oil, ¼ green chili, ¼ inch grated root ginger, pinch of chili powder, pinch of salt, ½ a large potato cut into chunks,  2oz of cauliflower cut into florets, 2oz okra trimmed and thickly sliced, 40ml natural low fat yogurt, 40ml vegetable stock, fresh coriander to garnish.

*Macros:  Protein: 8g   Carbs: 30g   Fat: 7.5g   Sodium: 1.1g*

*or*

**LOW** **Low Fat Aubergine Curry** - 1 medium aubergine approx. 100-120g, ¼ tablespoon of oil, pinch of black mustard seeds, 3 spring onions finel y chopped, 1oz button mushrooms halved, ½ garlic clove crushed, ¼ red chili finely chopped, pinch of chili powder, pinch of ground cumin, pinch of ground coriander, pinch of ground turmeric, pinch of salt, 100g or 1oz of chopped tomatoes, ¼ tablespoon fresh coriander, fresh coriander to garnish.

*Macros:  Protein: 8g   Carbs: 12g   Fat: 5.0g   Sodium: 1.2g*

*or*

**LOW** **Balti with Sweetcorn and Cauliflower** - Touch of oil, 1 curry leaf, pinch of onion seeds, half a chili seeded and chopped, 2oz of frozen or tinned sweetcorn, ¼ cauliflower cut into florets, 2 mint leaves.

*Macros:  Protein: 8g   Carbs: 20g   Fat: 4.5g   Sodium: 0.8g*

*or*

**LOW** **Low Fat Okra** - 125g of Okra, pinch of ground cumin, pinch of ground coriander, pinch of chili powder, pinch of ground turmeric, pinch of salt, pinch of sugar, squeeze of lemon juice, sprinkle of chopped fresh coriander, touch of oil, pinch of cumin seeds, pinch of mustard seeds, chopped fresh tomatoes to garnish.

*Macros:  Protein: 8g   Carbs: 10g   Fat: 5.0g    Sodium: 0.8g*

*or*

**HIGH** **Red Chillies with Potatoes** - 4-5 Baby New Potatoes peeled and halved, pinch of salt, touch of oil, pinch of crushed dried red chillies, pinch of cumin seeds, pinch of fennel seeds, pinch of crushed coriander seeds, 1 fresh red chili chopped (for milder version take out the seeds and disgard or use half a chili), pinch of fresh coriander.

*Macros:  Protein: 8g   Carbs: 30g   Fat: 4.0g    Sodium: 1.2g*

*or*

**LOW** **Vegetables with Almonds** – Touch of oil, ½ small onion sliced, ½ inch of root ginger shredded, pinch of crushed black peppercorns, pinch of ground turmeric, pinch of ground coriander, pinch of salt, 45g of mushrooms thickly sliced, ½ medium courgette thickly sliced, pinch of chopped fresh mint, 40ml of water, 1 tablespoon of natural low fat yogurt, flaked almonds to garnish.

*Macros:  Protein: 8g   Carbs: 10g   Fat: 11.3g    Sodium: 1.0g*

*or*

**HIGH** **Yogurt Covered Potatoes** – 1 medium baked potato chunked, 70g low fat natural yogurt, 75ml of water, pinch of ground turmeric, pinch of chili powder, pinch of ground coriander, pinch of ground cumin, pinch of salt, touch of oil, pinch of cumin seeds, pinch of chopped fresh coriander.

*Macros:  Protein: 10g   Carbs: 28g   Fat: 5.2g    Sodium: 1.2g*

## Supper Meals (Optional) This meal must be low carbohydrate

**H-L** **Soy, Hemp or Whey Protein Shake** - 2 scoops of Protein powder added to 200-300 ml of cold water or skimmed Milk

*Macros:  Protein: 40g   Carbs: 4g   Fat: 2.0g    Sodium: 0.4g*

*or*

**H-L** **Rice Cakes or Wholewheat Chapati** with 150-200g of low fat cottage cheese. *Macros: Protein: 20-25g  Carbs: 15g  Fat: 2.0g  Sodium: 1.0g*

*or*

**H-L** **Low Fat Cottage cheese** (200g) with Raspberries or gooseberries

*Macros: Protein: 25g  Carbs: 7g  Fat: 2.0g  Sodium: 1.0g*

*or*

**H-L** **Egg White Omelet** made with 5 egg whites, pepper, spinach and diced tomato (To increase the protein content add more egg whites. The white from a small egg = 4g of protein)

*Macros: Protein: 20g  Carbs: 10g  Fat: 2.0g  Sodium: 0.7g*

**Meal Extras:** You can add any of the following to your meal plans above if you need to increase carbohydrates.

## Beans

Soya Beans, Haricot Beans, Chickpeas, Black Beans, Kidney Beans, Butter Beans, White and Black Lentils and Cannelloni Beans. Avoid those in sauces or in salted water.

## Nuts and Seeds

Almonds, Brazil Nuts, Cashew Nuts, Pumpkin Seeds, Sunflower Seeds

## Greens

Lettuce, Spinach, Broccoli, Cauliflower, Cabbage, Asparagus

## Vitamins & Minerals

Vitamins are either water-soluble or fat-soluble. Water-soluble vitamins include vitamin B and C and are generally not stored in the body for more than a few hours, so their intake is very important. Fat soluble vitamins include A, D, E and K. These longer lasting vitamins will provide extended stimulus and will strongly decrease the chance of developing deficiencies.

## Water consumption

We all lose water every single minute of the day, when we walk, when we eat, and when we sleep. In the hot Indian climate during the hot summer weather we lose even more. Our body relies heavily on water and without it we would not survive. It produces energy, keeps us hydrated, regulates our body temperature, detoxifies our body and helps with numerous other functions. Do you often get headaches? feel irritable, low in energy or weak? If you answered yes, then your problem could very well stem from lack of water. So how much water do we need to maintain a healthy balance? You should ideally replenish your system with water every hour, keep a bottle of water with you at all times. A good way of checking your bodies hydration is to look at the color of your urine. Drink enough water to keep the color light yellow or clear. A golden/dark yellow coloring is a sign you're low on fluids and require replenishment. If you drink alcohol you should significantly increase water consumption as alcohol causes the body to lose even more water, replenishment is essential to dispose of the toxins found in alcohol.

# SUMMARY:

- Consume 5-6 smaller sized snack meals daily or 4 main meals and two shakes, it keeps your metabolism elevated – essential for fat loss!

- Be sure to see the Recipe pages for more meal ideas

- If you need to increase carbs in meals add any of the side dish recipes

- Drink water throughout the day.

- Eat plenty of green vegetables or green salad with your meals

- Avoid adding **excess oil or salt** to your cooking

- Food scales are very useful for measuring ingredients.

- Always try to oven cook or grill where possible

- If possible prepare some meals ahead of time and freeze or refrigerate. Many of the meals can be eaten cold, but with any rice dishes they should ideally be consumed within 24 hours.

# 'SIX-PACK' SUPERFOODS

Knowing what and what not to eat can be the most confusing aspect of any nutrition plan. Presented below is a list of the good and not so good foods which have been categorized to help you make better choices when preparing your meals. The 'Top 15' are the *best* foods to consume on a daily basis and should make up a large portion of your dietary intake. The 'Eat Often' category lists some more great foods that can be consumed throughout the week. The 'Eat Occasionally' foods should not be consumed more than once or twice weekly. Foods in the 'Eat Rarely' category should only be consumed on cheat days. Ok, let's take a look at the lists.

# TOP 15

- Almonds and Nuts
- All Indian Spices
- Beans, Lentils and Legumes
- Brown Basmati Rice
- Chicken / Lean Meats
- Egg Whites
- Dhal
- Fish (All Types) Tuna, Sardines, Cod, All White Fish etc.
- Green Vegetables, Spinach, Broccoli etc.
- Low Fat Cottage Cheese
- Lentils
- Idlis (Wholegrain or Brown Rice)
- Oats
- Olive Oil or Flaxseed Oil
- Raspberries and Gooseberries
- Soy or Tofu
- Wholegrain Cereal
- Whey Protein / Casein Protein Powder

# **EAT** OFTEN

- Apples
- Asparagus
- Avocado
- Bananas
- Brown Rice
- Baked Potato
- Canola Oil
- Citrus Fruit & Juices
- Coffee & Tea & Mossala Tea (No sugar)
- Green / Herbal Tea
- Granola
- Low Fat Spread
- Mushrooms
- Melon (All types)
- Peaches
- Peas & Beans
- Peppers
- Pumpkin Seeds
- Pine Nuts
- Sweet Potato
- Sunflower Seeds
- Sweetcorn / Corn on the cob
- Wholemeal / Wholegrain Pastas, Rice, Spaghetti

# **EAT** OCCASIONALLY

- Beer / Lager
- Chapati
- Dosas
- Non-Wholegrain Cereals
- Lamb (Remove fat)
- Luncheon Meat / Deli Ham
- Low Fat Ice Cream
- Potato Wedges
- Popcorn (Fat Free)
- Sugar Free Jams / Marmalade
- Soups
- Sugar Free Soda
- White Rice
- White Wine / Red Wine

# **EAT** RARELY

- Poppadoms
- Naan Breads
- Roti
- Burgers, Hot Dogs, Fast Food
- Chaat
- Chutney
- Candies / Jellies
- Creamer
- Creamed or Fried Vegetables
- Dosas
- Full Fat Peanut Butter
- Full Fat Milk
- Microwave / Processed Meals
- Ghee, Margarine or Butter
- Pooris / Bhatooras
- McDonald's, Pizza Hut, Dominos
- Pizza
- Potato Fries / Crisps
- Puddings and Cakes
- Paratha
- Pasta (Creamy)
- Soft Drinks High in Sugar
- Table Sugar
- Uttapams
- White Bread, Rolls

# Recommended
## Shopping List

Here's your shopping list which provides you with the recommended foods for the Program. Of course, you may not need all of the items listed. You may need additional items depending on your meal choices.

### SNACKS/SUPPLEMENTS

Whey Protein Powder or Soy Powder for vegetarians, available from Supplement Shops only.

### MEAT/POULTRY

Skinless chicken/turkey breasts or fresh breasts, Low-fat sliced chicken or turkey deli meat, Turkey burgers, Lean ground mutton, beef or steak, Ground turkey,

### GRAINS

Oats / Oatmeal, Whole-wheat tortillas, Idlis (Wholegrain or Brown Rice), Wholemeal Pita breads, Wholemeal bread or Rye Bread, Wholemeal buns/rolls, Wholemeal spaghetti/pasta, Wholemeal flour, Rice Cakes (Oat Bran or Flavored Variety), Granola, Kashi, Bran Flakes, Shredded Wheat or other Wholegrain Cereal, Brown Basmati Rice, Wholegrain Rice.

### VEGETABLES

Aubergines, Broccoli, Celery, Cauliflower, Okra, Water Chestnuts,

Spinach leaves, Fresh tomatoes, Cucumber, Carrots, Romaine Lettuce, Broccoli, Sweet Potatoes, White Potatoes, Lettuce, Onions, Canned Whole Tomatoes, Fresh Mushrooms, Corn on the Cob, Sweetcorn, Red Kidney Beans

## SPICES

Bay Leaves, Cardamom Pods, Cinnamon, Chillies, Chili Powder, Cloves, Coriander leaves, seeds and powder, Curry Leaves, Cumin, Curry Powder, Fennel Seeds, Fenugreek Fresh and seeds, Garam Masala, Garlic Cloves and Granules, Ginger, Mint, Mustard Seeds, Nutmeg, Onion Seeds, Paprika, Pepper, Peppercorns, Poppy Seeds, Saffron, Sesame Seeds, Tamarind, Turmeric

## LENTILS

Black-eyed beans, Chickpeas, Chana Dhal, Haricot Beans, Kidney Beans, Masoor Dhal, Moong Dhal, Mung Beans, Toor Dhal, Urid Dhal

## OILS/DRESSINGS

Extra virgin olive oil, Balsamic vinaigrette, Low-fat mayonnaise or low fat salad cream, Cooking spray

## FRUIT/NUTS

Blueberries, Gooseberries, Raspberries, Apples, Apricots, Bananas, Peaches, Melon, Pears

## SEEDS

Pumpkin Seeds, Soy Nuts, Sesame Seeds, Linseeds, Hemp Seeds, Sunflower Seeds, Mixed Nuts, Almonds, Brazil Nuts, Cashews, Peanuts etc.

## DAIRY

Low Fat Fromage Frais, Low-fat cheese slices, low-fat American cheese, Skimmed milk, Low-fat cottage cheese, Fresh eggs, Low-fat yogurt

## FISH

All types of fresh or frozen fish, Canned Tuna, Cod, Hake, Monkfish and all White Fish, Trout, Canned Salmon, Salmon Fillet, Haddock

## TOPPINGS/CONDIMENTS

Sugar-free syrup, Fresh lime juice, Almonds/slivered almonds, All-natural peanut butter, Green enchilada sauce, Salsa, Light Soy sauce, Lime juice, Apple sauce, Baking powder, Lemon juice, Ketchup, Cranberry Sauce, Dijon mustard

## DRINKS

Tea, Green Tea, Mossala Tea or Coffee, Bottled Water,
Sugar Free Soda (Should not replace water) Drink Occasionally
Fresh Fruit Juice (100% Freshly Squeezed) Drink Occasionally
Cranberry Juice (Drink Occasionally)

# **Recipes** Meat & Fish

*All meals serve 1 person, simply double ingredients to serve 2.*
*With all meat, fish, amount mentioned in grams refers to uncooked*
*weight*

## **Egg White Omelette**     Top Choice ✓     Low Carb
Nutritional Facts: Protein 25g, Carbs 4g, Saturated Fat 2.5g, Unsaturated Fat 4g

*Ingredients:*
8 egg whites, 2 yolks, 1 teaspoon of oil, 1 small onion chopped, 5 button
mushrooms, ½ green or red pepper, white or black pepper to taste

*Add to this meal?*
Chapati, Rice

*Preparation*: First separate the yolks from the whites and disgard six of the
yolks. Chop the onions and mushrooms into smaller pieces along with the
pepper. With a frying pan heat a touch of oil. First add the vegetables and fry
for approximately 1-2 minutes, then stir in the eggs until they set. Add a little oil
to the sides and flip to cook other side.

## **Microwaved Omelette**     Top Choice ✓     Low Carb
Nutritional Facts: Protein 25g, Carbs 4g, Saturated Fat 3.5g, Unsaturated Fat 4g

*Ingredients:*
8 egg whites, 2 yolks, 1 teaspoon of oil, 1 small onion chopped, 2 green chillies
finely chopped, few sprigs of fresh coriander, 1 tablespoon of milk, pepper to
taste, 1 tablespoon of butter or low fat spread

*Add to this meal?*
Chapati, Rice

*Preparation*: Beat the eggs (8 whites and 2 yolks) and stir in the chopped onions,
chillies, coriander, milk and pepper. Place one tablespoon of butter or low fat
spread in a flat microwave dish and cook uncovered for 20 seconds. Spread the
melted butter evenly and then pour in the omelette mixture ensuring that it
spreads evenly. Cook uncovered on high for 3 minutes. Leave to stand for one
minute.

## Chicken Tikka — Top Choice ✓ — Low Carb

Nutritional Facts: Protein 30g, Carbs 4g, Saturated Fat 1.5g, Unsaturated Fat 4g

*Ingredients:*
200g of boneless chicken breast, skinned and cubed, ¼ tsp of ginger pulp, ¼ tsp of garlic pulp, ¼ tsp of chili powder, pinch of turmeric, pinch of salt, 40ml of natural low fat yogurt, ¼ tablespoon of lemon juice, chopped fresh coriander, ¼ tablespoon of oil
*For Garnish:*
Mixed Salad Leaves, 1 small onion cut into rings, lime wedges (Optional), fresh coriander

*Add to this meal?*
Chapati, Rice

*Preparation*: First add the chicken, ginger, garlic, chili, turmeric, salt, yogurt, lime juice and coriander in a medium bowl and leave to marinade for 2 hours.

Place in a grill pan or dish and baste with a little oil. Grill the chicken for 15-20 minutes. Serve on a bed of mixed salad leaves or Chapati, Rice depending on low or high carb day.

## Tandoori Chicken — Low Carb

Nutritional Facts: Protein 30g, Carbs 6g, Saturated Fat 3.5g, Unsaturated Fat 7g

*Ingredients:*
200g of boneless chicken breast, skinned and cut into sizeable chunks, ¼ tsp garam masala, ¼ tsp of ginger pulp, ¼ tsp of garlic pulp, ¼ tsp of chili powder, pinch of turmeric, pinch of salt, 50ml of natural low fat yogurt, ¼ tablespoon of lemon juice, chopped fresh coriander, ¼ tablespoon of oil

*For Garnish:*
Mixed Salad Leaves, 1 small onion cut into rings, lime wedges (Optional), fresh coriander

*Add to this meal?*
Chapati, Rice

*Preparation*: Rinse and pat dry the chicken, take off any remaining fat. Make two deep slits in flesh of the breast. Place is dish and set aside. Then mix together the yogurt, garam masala, ginger, garlic, chili powder, turmeric, coriander, lemon juice, salt and optional red food colouring and then beat so that the ingredients are combined. Add a touch of oil if needed.

Cover the chicken with spice mixture and leave to marinate for three hours. Pre-heat oven to Gas Mark 9 (240 degrees) and place the chicken in overproof dish. Bake the chicken in overn for 20-25 minutes. When cooked serve with salad.

## Balti Chicken Vindaloo          Top Choice ✓
Nutritional Facts: Protein 30g, Carbs 20g, Saturated Fat 0.5g, Unsaturated Fat 3.5g

*Ingredients:*
1 large potato, 200g of boneless chicken breast, 40ml malt vinegar,  ½ tablespoon crushed coriander seeds, ¼ tsp crushed cumin seeds, ½ tsp chili powder, ¼ tsp of ginger pulp, ¼ tsp of garlic pulp, pinch of salt, ½ tablespoon of paprika, ¼ tablespoon tomato puree, 100ml water, touch of oil, 1 medium onion sliced, 1 curry leaf, 1 green chili chopped

*Add to this meal?*
Chapati, Rice

*Preparation*: Peel the potato and cut into large irregular shapes, place in bowl of water and set aside. Mix together the vinegar, coriander, cumin, chili powder, turmeric, garlic, ginger, salt, paprika, tomato puree, fenugreek and water. Then, pour the mixture over the chicken and set aside.
Heat a touch of oil in a wok or deep pan and fry the onion and curry leaf, without burning. Then, lower the heat and add the chicken mixture, continue to stir fry for a further 2 minutes. Drain the potato pieces and add to the pan. Cover with a lid and cook for an additional 5-7 minutes or until the sauce has thickened and the chicken and potatoes are cooked through. Add the chopped green chillies before serving.

## Tandoori Masala Spring Lamb          Low Carb
Nutritional Facts: Protein 25g, Carbs 4g, Saturated Fat 2.5g, Unsaturated Fat 4g

*Ingredients:*
150-200g of diced lamb (cut fat where possible), ½ tablespoon of low fat yogurt, ¼ tablespoon tomato puree, ½ tsp ground coriander, ¼ tsp ginger pulp, ¼ tsp garlic pulp, ¼ tsp chili powder, ¼ tsp of salt, ¼ tablespoon of oil, 1 tablespoon of lemon juice

*For Garnish:*
Lettuce Leaves, Lime Wedges (Optional), 1 small onion sliced, fresh coriander

*Add to this meal?*
Chapati, Rice

*Preparation:* Trim any excess fat from the meat. Then in a medium bowl mix together the yogurt, ground coriander, tomato puree, ginger and garlic pulp, chili powder, salt, oil and lemon juice. Then rub this mixture over the lamb and leave to marinade for three hours.

Preheat the oven at Gas Mark 8 and place the marinated lamb in an ovenproof dish into the oven and cook for 10 minutes. Lower the heat to Gas Mark 4 and cook in the oven for 10 minutes

## Prawns with Vegetables                                    Low Carb
Nutritional Facts: Protein 25g, Carbs 5g, Saturated Fat 1.4g, Unsaturated Fat 6g

*Ingredients:*
8 King Prawns Peeled, ½ tablespoon chopped fresh coriander, 1 Green chili, 1 tablespoon of lemon juice, ¾ tablespoon of oil, 1 medium courgette sliced, 1 medium onion cut into chunks, some cherry tomatoes, 3 baby corn on the cobs

*For Garnish:*
Mixed Salad Leaves

*Add to this meal?*
Chapati, Rice

Heat a touch of oil in a wok or deep pan, add all ingredients except prawns and stir fry for 5 minutes. Then add prawns and fry for additional 4 minutes.

## Pineapple Chicken Kebabs
Nutritional Facts: Protein 30g, Carbs 15g, Saturated Fat 1.5g, Unsaturated Fat 5g

*Ingredients:*
200g of boneless chicken, skinned and cubed, 60g of canned pineapple, ¼ tsp ground cumin, ¼ tsp ground coriander, ¼ tsp chili powder, ¼ tsp garlic pulp, ¼ tsp salt, ½ tablespoon natural low fat yogurt, ½ tablespoon of chopped fresh coriander, ¼ of yellow or green pepper seeded, ½ an onion, 2 cherry tomatoes, ¼ tablespoon of oil

*For Garnish:*
Mixed Salad Leaves

*Add to this meal?*
Chapati, Rice

*Preparation:* Drain pineapple into a bowl, reserve a few chunks and then drain the juice into a bowl and set aside. Then in a large bowl , blend together the spices, garlic, salt, yogurt and fresh coriander, mix in the reserved pineapple juice.

Cut the chicken into bite sized cubes, add to the mixture you just prepared and leave to marinate in a cool place for 1-2 hours.

Cut the onion and peppers into bite sized chunks. Arrange the chicken, onion and peppers onto skewers and grill on a medium heat for 15-20 minutes. Brush the kebabs with a touch of oil. Another quick and easy protein packed meal!

## Lamb with Peas and Mint          Low Carb
Nutritional Facts: Protein 25g, Carbs 8g, Saturated Fat 3g, Unsaturated Fat 6g

*Ingredients:*
150-200g of lamb minced, ¼ medium onion chopped, ¼ tsp garlic pulp, ¼ tsp root ginger pulp, ¼ tsp chili powder, ¼ tsp ground coriander, pinch of salt, 1 medium tomato sliced, ½ a large carrot sliced, ¼ cup fo petit pois, ¼ tablespoon fresh mint, ¼ tablespoon chopped fresh coriander, ½ green chili chopped, fresh coriander to garnish

*Add to this meal?*
Chapati, Rice, Bombay Potato

*Preparation:* In a deep frying pan, heat the oil and fry the chopped onion for five minutes. In a small mixing bowl, blend together the garlic, ginger, chili powder, turmeric, ground coriander and salt,

Add the sliced tomato and spice mixture to the onions and fry for a further 2-3 minutes stirring continuously. Then add the minced lamb and cook for a further 8-10 minutes. Finally add the carrot, peas, fresh mint, coriander and chili mix and stir fy for a further 2-3 minutes.

## Stir Fry Lamb with Baby Onions and Peppers     Low Carb

Nutritional Facts: Protein 25g, Carbs 6g, Saturated Fat 3g, Unsaturated Fat 6g

*Ingredients:*
150-200g of lamb cut into strips, ¼ tablespoon of oil, 2 baby onions, ¼ tsp of ground cumin, ¼ tsp ground coriander, ¼ tablespoon tomato puree, ¼ tsp chili powder, pinch of salt, pinch of lemon, ¼ tsp onion seeds, 1 curry leaf, 100ml of water, half a red pepper, ¼ tablespoon chopped fresh coriander, ¼ tablespoon chopped fresh mint

*Add to this meal?*
Chapati, Rice, Bombay Potato

*Preparation*: Heat a touch of oil in a deep pan or wok and then fry the baby onions for 3 minutes. Once done, drain and set aside. Then mix together the lamb, cumin, ground coriander, tomato puree, chili powder, salt and lemon juice in a bowl and set aside.

In the same pan you fried the onions, now gently fry the curry leaves and onion seeds for 2-3 minutes. Then add the lamb mixture and stir fry for about 5 minutes, then add in the water and lower the heat to cook for around 7-10 minutes. Add the peppers and half the fresh mint and coriander and stir fry for a further 2 minutes. Finally add the baby onions for another 1 minute.

## Lamb Meatballs     Low Carb

Nutritional Facts: Protein 25g, Carbs 6g, Saturated Fat 5g, Unsaturated Fat 7g

*Ingredients for the meatballs:*
175g lean ground lamb mince, ¼ green chili roughly chopped, ¼ of a garlic clove chopped, ¼ inch of root ginger chopped, 0.5ml garam masala, pinch of salt, 1 tablespoon fresh coriander chopped,

*Ingredients for the Sauce:*
¼ tablespoon of oil, cumin seeds (¼ tsp), half an onion chopped, ¼ clove of garlic chopped, ¼ inch of root ginger chopped, ¼ tsp ground cumin, ¼ tsp ground coriander, pinch of salt, pinch of chili powder, ¼ tablespoon tomato puree, 100g of chopped tomatoes

*Add to this meal?*
Chapati, Rice

*Preparation*: Blend all the ingredients in a blender, then shape the mixture into balls, cover and chill for 10 minutes. To make the sauce, heat a little oil in a deep pan and pan fry the cumin seends until they splutter. Add the onion, garlic and ginger and stir fry for 5 minutes. Stir in the remaining ingredients and simmer for 5 minutes.

Add the meatballs to the sauce, bring to the boil, cover and simmer for 15-20 minutes until meatballs are cooked through.

## Courgettes with Lamb    Top Choice ✓    Low Carb
Nutritional Facts: Protein 25g, Carbs 10g, Saturated Fat 2.5g, Unsaturated Fat 5.5g

*Ingredients:*
150-175g of lamb steaks cut into strips, ¼ tablespoon of oil, 1 medium onion chopped, 40ml (¼ cup) of natural low fat yogurt, ¼ tsp garam masala, ¼ tsp chili powder, ¼ tsp garlic pulp, ¼ tsp ginger pulp, ¼ tsp ground coriander, 1 medium courgette, add fresh coriander to garnish

*Add to this meal?*
Chapati, Rice

*Preparation*: Heat the oil in a wok and fry onions until golden. Add the lamb strips and stir fry for 1 minute. Put the Yogurt, Garam Masala, chili Powder, Garlic, Ginger and Ground Coriander into a bowl and mix together.

Then pour that mixture over the lamb and cook for a further 2 minutes. Cover and then gently cook on low heat for 10-15 minutes. Grill the courgettes pieces under grill for 2 minutes on each side. Then add the courgettes into lamb towards the end of cooking time.

## Balti Lamb with Cauliflower
Nutritional Facts: Protein 25g, Carbs 10g, Saturated Fat 3.2g, Unsaturated Fat 6g

*Ingredients:*
150-175g of lamb steaks cut into strips, ½ tsp of oil, 1 medium onion sliced, ½ tsp ginger pulp, ¼ tsp chili powder, ¼ tsp garlic pulp, pinch of ground turmeric, pinch of ground coriander, 1 tablespoon of fresh fenugreek leaves, ½ small cauliflower cut into small florets, 100ml of water, ½ tablespoon fresh coriander leaves, ¼ red pepper, ¼ tablespoon of lemon juice

*Add to this meal?*
Chapati, Rice, Bombay Potato

*Preparation*: First, gently fry the onions in a little oil until golden brown. Then, lower the heat and add in the ginger pulp, chili powder, garlic pulp, turmeric and ground coriander. Stir well and the add the fenugreek leaves.

Add the lamb strips and stir fry, also add the cauliflower florets. Pour in the water, cover and cook on a low heat for 5-7 minutes. Then add half the fresh coriander, red pepper and lemon juice and stiry fry for about 3 minutes. Make sure the sauce does not stick so keep stirring.

To make the Tarka, heat the oil and fry the seeds and leave for 30 seconds. While it is still hot pour it over the lamb.

## Spiced Lamb with Chillies                      Low Carb
Nutritional Facts: Protein 30g, Carbs 10g, Saturated Fat 2.7g, Unsaturated Fat 5.7g

*Ingredients:*
4-5oz lean lamb fillet, 40ml natural low fat yogurt, pinch of ground cardamom, ¼ tsp ginger pulp, ¼ tsp garlic pulp, ¼ tsp chili powder, ¼ tsp garam masala, pinch of salt, ¼ tablespoon of oil, 1 medium onion chopped, 1 bay leaf, 100ml of water, 1 green chili sliced lengthways, 1 red chili sliced lengthways, 1 tablespoon of fresh coriander leaves

*Add to this meal?*
Chapati, Rice, Bombay Potato

*Preparation*: Remove any fat from the lamb and cut into even sized strips. Mix together the yogurt, cardamom, ginger pulp, garlic pulp, chili powder, garam masala and salt.Add the lamb and leave for about 1 hour to marinate.

Heat a touch of oil in a wok or heavy based frying pan and fry onion for 3-5 minutes. Add the lamb with the yogurt and spice mixture and stir fry for 2-3 minutes over a medium heat. Then pour over the water, cover and cook for 15 minutes over a low heat. Once the water has evaporated, stir fry for a further minute. Add the chillies and coriander and serve hot.

## Balti Beef                                                    Low Carb

Nutritional Facts: Protein 30g, Carbs 8g, Saturated Fat 4.5g, Unsaturated Fat 7g

*Ingredients:*
200g lean rump or fillet steak, ½ red or green pepper, ¼ tablespoon of oil, ¼ tsp cumin seeds, pinch of fennel seeds, ½ onion cut into wedges, ¼ garlic clove crushed, ¼ inch of root ginger finely chopped, ¼ tablespoon of curry paste, pinch of salt

*Add to this meal?*
Chapati, Rice, Bombay Potato

*Preparation:* First cut the peppers into chunks. Heat a touch of oil in a frying pan and add the cumin and fennel seeds for about 2 minutes until they splutter. Add the garlic, onion, ginger and chili and stir fry for a further 5 minutes.

Add the curry paste and salt and fry for a further 3 minutes. Then, add the peppers and fry for a further 4 minutes. Stir in the beef strips and fry for a further 8 minutes or until meat is to your liking.


## Beef with Green Beans Stir Fry                              Low Carb

Nutritional Facts: Protein 30g, Carbs 9g, Saturated Fat 3.0g, Unsaturated Fat 7g

*Ingredients:*
200g lean beef cubed, 60g of green beans cut into pieces, ¼ tablespoon of oil, ½ a medium onion sliced, ¼ tsp of ginger pulp, ¼ tsp of garlic pulp, ¼ tsp chili powder, pinch of salt, pinch of turmeric, 1 tomato chopped, ½ a red pepper sliced and seeded, ¼ tablespoon of fresh coriander, 1 green chili chopped,

*Add to this meal?*
Chapati, Rice, Bombay Potato

*Preparation:* Blanch the beans in boiling water for 3 minutes. Then rinse and drain and set aside. Heat a touch of oil in a heavy based pan or wok and gently fry the onion until golden. Mix together the ginger pulp, garlic pulp, chili powder, salt, turmeric and chopped tomatoes. Put mixture into onion and fry for further few minutes. Add the beef and stir fry for 3 minutes. When done add the green beans. Finally add the pepper, fresh coriander and chillies and fry for fuerther 3 minutes. Quick and easy!

## Chicken Korma                                          Low Carb

Nutritional Facts: Protein 30g, Carbs 10g, Saturated Fat 2.5g, Unsaturated Fat 7g

*Ingredients:*
200g of chicken breast, skinned and cubed, ½ garlic clove crushed, ¼ inch piece of root ginger roughly chopped, ¼ tablespoon of oil, 1 green cardamom pod, ½ onion finely chopped, 1/3 tsp of ground cumin, pinch of salt, 80ml of natural low fat yogurt

*Add to this meal?*
Chapati, Rice, Bombay Potato

*Preparation*: Remove any fat from chicken breasts and cut into cubes. Blend the garlic and ginger adding a little water to make paste. Heat a touch of oil in wok or heavy based pan and cook chicken cubes for 8-10 minutes, then remove and set aside.

Add the cardamom pods and fry for 2 minutes, add the onion and fry for a further 5 minutes. Stir in garlic and ginger paste, cumin and salt and cook for a further 5 minutes. Add half the yogurt, stirring in a tablespoonful at a time and cook over a low heat until it has been absorbed. Return the chicken to the pan. Cover and simmer for 5 minutes. Add the remaining yogurt and simmer for a further 5 minutes. Garnish with flaked almonds and coriander (optional).

## Balti Chicken Madras                    Top Choice ✓

Nutritional Facts: Protein 30g, Carbs 10g, Saturated Fat 0.5g, Unsaturated Fat 3.6g

*Ingredients:*
200g of chicken breast, skinned and cubed, 1 tablespoon tomato puree, pinch of fennel seeds, ¼ tsp ginger pulp, ½ tsp ground coriander, ¼ tsp garlic pulp, ¼ tsp chili powder, pinch of ground turmeric, ½ tablespoon of lemon juice, pinch of salt, 80ml of water (¼ of a cup), ¼ tablespoon of oil, ½ a medium onion diced, 1 curry leave, 1 green chili, seeded and chopped, fresh coriander leaves to top.

*Add to this meal?*
Chapati, Rice, Bombay Potato

*Preparation:* Remove any fat from chicken and cut breast meat into cubes. Then mix the tomato puree, fennel seeds, ginger, coriander, garlic, chili powder, turmeric, lemon juice, salt and water into a mixing bowl.

Heat small amount of oil in a wok or deep frying pan and fry the onions together with curry leaves until brown. Then add the chicken pieces and stir fry for about 1 minute to seal the chicken. Then, add the spice mixture and continue to stir fry for a further 2 minutes. Lower the heat and cook for 8-10 minutes.

## Balti Chicken Curry — Low Carb

Nutritional Facts: Protein 30g, Carbs 10g, Saturated Fat 2.5g, Unsaturated Fat 7g

*Ingredients:*
200g of chicken breast, skinned and cubed, ¼ tablespoon of oil, pinch of cumin seeds, pinch of fennel seeds, ½ an onion thickly sliced, ½ a crushed garlic clove, ¼ of an inch of root ginger finely chopped, ¼ tablespoon of curry paste, 1 tomato cut into wedges, 2 oz or 50g of broccoli broken into florets, ¼ tsp of garam masala, fresh coriander to top

*Add to this meal?*
Chapati, Rice, Bombay Potato

*Preparation:* Remove any fat from chicken and cut breast meat into cubes.

Heat small amount of oil in a wok or deep frying pan and fry the fennel and cumin seeds for 2 minutes until the seeds begin to splutter. Add the onion, garlic, giner and cook for 5-7 minutes. Stir in curry paste and cook for an additional 2 minutes. Next, add the broccoli florets and fry for approximately 4-5 minutes, then, add the chicken cubes and cook for 8 minutes.

## Balti Chicken in Hara Masala Sauce — Top Choice ✓

Nutritional Facts: Protein 30g, Carbs 15g, Saturated Fat 2g, Unsaturated Fat 3.0g

*Ingredients:*
200g of chicken breast, skinned and cubed, ½ a green apple peeled, cored and cut into cubes, 1tablespoon of fresh coriander leaves, ½ tablespoon of fresh mint leaves, 40 ml of natural low fat yogurt, 1 tablespoon of low fat fromage frais, 1 medium chili seeded and chopped, handful of spring onions chopped, pinch of salt, pinch of sugar, ¼ tsp of garlic pulp, ¼ tsp of ginger pulp, tsp of oil, 10g of sultanas

*Add to this meal?*
Chapati, Rice, Bombay Potato

*Preparation:* Remove any fat from chicken and cut breast meat into cubes. Place the apple, coriander, mint, fromage frais, chillies, yogurt, onions, garlic, and ginger into a blender and blend for one minute.

Heat the oil in a wok or deep frying pan and pour in the mixture and cook on a low heat for 2 minutes. Then, add the chicken pieces and blend together. Cook on a low heat for 10-15 minutes. Finally, add sultanas and fresh coriander leaves.

## Balti Chicken in Thick Creamy Coconut Sauce   Low Carb
Nutritional Facts: Protein 30g, Carbs 7g, Saturated Fat 3g, Unsaturated Fat 8g

*Ingredients:*
200g of chicken breast, skinned and cubed, ¼ tablespoon ground almonds, ¼ tablespoon of dessicated coconut, 20ml coconut milk, 45g or 2oz of low fat fromage frais, ½ tsp of ground coriander, ¼ tsp chili powder, ¼ tsp garlic pulp, ½ tsp ginger pulp, pinch of salt, ¼ tablespoon of oil, 1 green cardamom pod, bay leaf or curry leaf (optional), 1.4 of a dried red chili crushed fresh coriander to top

*Add to this meal?*
Chapati, Rice, Bombay Potato

Using a wok or deep frying pan dry roast the ground almonds and coconut until they turn slightly darker. Then, add the coconut milk, fromage frais, ground coriander, chili powder, garlic, ginger and salt into a mixing bowl.

Heat a small amount of oil in wok or deep frying pan and add the chicken cubes, cardamoms and bay leaf. Fry for 2 minutes just to seal the chicken pieces. Then, pour in the coconut mixture, lower the heat, add the fresh coriander and chili, cover and cook for 10 minutes stirring occassionally.

## Balti Chicken in Orange and Black Pepper Sauce
Nutritional Facts: Protein 30g, Carbs 15g, Saturated Fat 1.5g, Unsaturated Fat 5g

*Ingredients:*
200g of chicken breast, skinned and cubed, 50g or 2oz of low fat fromage frais, 15ml of natural low fat yogurt, 40ml of orange juice, ½ tsp of ginger pulp, ¼ tsp of garlic pulp, ¼ tsp of ground black pepper, pinch of salt, ¼ tsp ground

coriander, ¼ tablespoon of oil, 1 bay leaf or curry leaf, ½ an onion chopped, fresh mint leaves, ¼ green chili, seeded and chopped

*Add to this meal?*
Chapati, Rice, Bombay Potato

*Preparation:* Using a mixing bowl whisk together the fromage frais, yogurt, orange juice, ginger, garlic, pepper, salt and coriander, then pour this over the chicken and leave for 3-4 hours.

Heat a small amount of oil with a bay leaf in wok or deep frying pan and fry the onion until soft. Pour in the chicken mixture and stir fry for 3-4 minutes over a medium heat. Then, lower the heat, cover and cook for an additional 8 minutes. If the sauce is too thick just add a little water.

## Karahi Chicken with Mint                                Low Carb
Nutritional Facts: Protein 30g, Carbs 5g, Saturated Fat 2g, Unsaturated Fat 6g

*Ingredients:*
200g of chicken breast, skinned and cut into strips, 75ml of water, ½ tablespoon of oil, 2 spring onions chopped, ¼ tsp of shredded root ginger, ¼ tsp of crushed dried chillies, ¾ tablespoon of lemon juice, ¼ tablespoon chopped fresh coriander, ¼ tablespoon chopped fresh mint, 1 tomato skinned, seeded and roughly chopped, pinch of salt, mint, coriander to garnish

*Add to this meal?*
Chapati, Rice, Potato

Place the chicken and water into a saucepan, bringing to the boil and then lower the heat to medium. Cook for approximately 10 minutes or until water has evaporated and chicken is cooked.

Heat a small amount of oil in a wok or deep frying pan and stir fry the spring onions for about 2 minutes until soft. Add the boiled chicken and stir fry for a further 3 minutes over medium heat. Gradually add the shredded ginger, red chillies, lemon juice, chopped coriander and mint, tomatoes and salt.

## Tandoori Chicken Kebabs    Top Choice ✓   Low Carb

Nutritional Facts: Protein 30g, Carbs 4g, Saturated Fat 2g, Unsaturated Fat 6g

*Ingredients:*
200g of chicken breast, skinned and cubed, ¼ tablespoon of lemon juice, 1 tablespoon of tandoori paste, 1 tablespoon of low fat yogurt, ¼ garlic clove crushed, ½ tablespoon of freshly chopped coriander, pinch of salt and black pepper, ½ an onion cut into wedges and separated into layers, a little oil brushed, fresh corainder sprigs to garnish

*Add to this meal?*
Chapati, Rice, Potato

*Preparation:* Chop the chicken breasts into cubes, place in a mixing bowl and add the lemon juice, tandoori paste, yogurt, garlic, chopped coriander and seasoning. Cover and leave to marinade for 2-3 hours.

With grill on high, thread the chicken cubes onto a skewer along with slices of onion inbetween each piece of chicken. Brush the skewers with a little oil and place on grill for 10-12 minutes turning to ensure both sides are cooked.


## Balti Chicken with Panir and Peas      Low Carb

Nutritional Facts: Protein 30g, Carbs 4g, Saturated Fat 4.5g, Unsaturated Fat 5g

*Ingredients:*
200g of chicken breast, skinned and cubed, ½ tablespoon of tomato puree, 1 tablespoon of low fat yogurt, ¼ tsp of garam masala, ¼ tsp of garlic pulp, ¼ tsp of ginger pulp, ¼ tablespoon of chili powder, pinch of salt, pinch of sugar, ½ tsp of oil, ¼ inch of cinnamon stick, ½ black peppercorn, 75ml of water, 1oz or 30g of panir, cubed, ½ tablespoon of fresh coriander leaves, ½ green chili seeded and chopped, 20g or 1oz peas

*Add to this meal?*
Chapati, Rice, Potato

*Preparation:* Skin the chicken and cut into squares. Using a mixing bowl add the tomato puree, yogurt, garam masala, garlic pulp, ginger pulp, cardamom, chili powder, turmeric, salt and sugar.

Heat a little oil in a wok or deep frying pan. Add the spices and mixture from above. Lower the heat and cook gently for 3 minutes, then pour in water and bring to simmer. Add the chicken pieces and stir fry for 2 minutes, then cover the pan and cook over medium heat for 8 minutes.

Then, add the panir cubes to the pan, followed by half the coriander and half the green chillies, Mix together and cook for a further 5 minutes. Finally, stir in the fromage frais and peas and heat through for a minute before serving.

## Chicken Balti with Spicy Lentil Sauce
Nutritional Facts: Protein 30g, Carbs 20g, Saturated Fat 1.5g, Unsaturated Fat 6g

*Ingredients:*
200g of chicken breast, skinned and cubed, ½ tablespoon of chana dhal, 15g or 1oz of masoor dhal, ¼ tablespoon of oil, 1 medium onion chopped, ¼ tsp garlic pulp, ¼ tsp ginger pulp, pinch of ground turmeric, ½ tsp of chili powder, ¼ tsp of garam masala, pinch of ground coriander, pinch of salt, 1 tablespoon of fresh coriander leaves, ½ green chili, seeded and chopped, 1 tablespoon of lemon juice, 75ml of water, 1 tomato peeled and halved

*Add to this meal?*
Chapati, Rice, Potato

Boil both the chana dhal and masoor dhal together in a saucepan until soft and mushy, then set aside for later.

Heat a little oil in a wok or deep frying pan and fry the onions until golden brown. Stir in the garlic, turmeric, chili powder, garam masala, ground coriander and salt. Then, add chicken pieces and stir fry for 5 minutes to seal the meat.

Add half the fresh coriander, green chillies, water and lemon juice and cook for an additional 4 minutes before adding in the chana and masoor dhal. Add the coriander.

# King Prawn Korma                                          Low Carb
Nutritional Facts: Protein 25g, Carbs 8g, Saturated Fat 1g, Unsaturated Fat 5g

*Ingredients:*
5 king prawns thawed and peeled, 1 tablespoon of nautral low fat yogurt, 1 tablespoon of low fat fromage frais, ¼ tsp of ground paprika, ¼ tsp garam masala, ¼ tablespoon tomato puree, 1 tablespoon coconut milk, ¼ tablespoon chili powder, 40ml of water, ¼ tablespoon of oil, ¼ tsp of ginger pulp, ¼ tsp of garlic pulp, ½ green cardamom pod, pinch of salt, chopped fresh coriander to garnish

*Add to this meal?*
Chapati, Rice, Potato

*Preparation:* Drain the prawns. Place yogurt, fromage frais, garam masala, paprika, tomato puree, chili powder, coconut milk and water in a mixing bowl and blend all ingredients together, then set aside.

Heat a little oil in a wok or deep pan, add the garlic, ginger, cinnamon, cardamoms and salt and fry over low heat. Then, turn up the heat and add the mixture bringing to the boil. Add the prawns and continue to stir fry until sauce is thick and prawns cooked.

# Prawn and Vegetable Balti                                  Low Carb
Nutritional Facts: Protein 25g, Carbs 10g, Saturated Fat 1.5g, Unsaturated Fat 6.5g

*Ingredients:*
5 king prawns thawed and peeled or 125-150g of peeled prawns, ½ tablespoon of oil, pinch of onion seeds, 1-2 curry leaves, 35g of frozen peas, 35g of sweetcorn, ½ a courgette sliced, ½ a medium red pepper, seeded and roughly sliced, ¼ tsp crushed coriander seeds, ¼ tsp crushed dried red chillies, pinch of salt, ¼ tablespoon of lemon juice, fresh coriander leaves to garnish

*Add to this meal?*
Chapati, Rice, Potato

Heat a little oil in a wok or deep frying pan. Add the onion seeds and curry leaves. Then, add the prawns. Next, add the peas, sweetcorn, courgette and red pepper and stir fry for 4 minutes. Finally, add the crushed coriander seeds and chillies with pinch of salt and lemon juice to taste.

## Grilled King Prawn Bhoona   Top Choice ✓   Low Carb
Nutritional Facts: Protein 30g, Carbs 15g, Saturated Fat 0.5g, Unsaturated Fat 3.5g

*Ingredients:*
5-6 king prawns thawed and peeled or 125-150g of peeled prawns, ¼ tsp paprika, ¼ tsp ginger pulp, pinch of salt, 1 tablespoon of natural low fat yogurt, ¼ tablespoon of oil, 1 medium onion sliced, pinch of fennel seeds crushed, ¼ piece of cinnamon bark (optional), ¼ tsp garlic pulp, ¼ tsp chili powder, 1/3 a yellow or red pepper seeded and roughly chopped, fresh coriander leaves to garnish

*Add to this meal?*
Chapati, Rice, Potato

*Preparation:* In a mixing bowl mix together the yogurt, ginger, paprika and pinch of salt. Pour the mixture over the prawns and leave to marinade for 30-45 minutes.

Using a wok or deep frying pan add a touch of oil and fry the onions with the fennel seeds. Lower the heat and add the garlic and chili powder. Then, add the peppers and stir fry gently for 3-4 minutes. Remove from heat and transfer to serving dish. For chargrilled taste place prawns under grill for 3 minutes.

## King Prawns with Onion and Curry Leaves   Low Carb
Nutritional Facts: Protein 25g, Carbs 8g, Saturated Fat 1g, Unsaturated Fat 5g

*Ingredients:*
5 king prawns thawed and peeled or 125-150g of peeled prawns, 1 medium onion, ¼ tablespoon of oil, 2 curry leaves, pinch of onion seeds, ¼ of a green chili seeded and diced, ¼ tsp shredded root ginger, pinch of salt, ¼ tablespoon of fresh fenugreek leaves

*Add to this meal?*
Chapati, Rice, Potato

Cut the onions into thin slices. Heat a little oil in wok or deep frying pan and fry the onions with curry leaves and onion seeds for 2-3 minutes. Then, add the chillies, followed by prawns and cook for a further 5-6 minutes, adding ginger and pinch of salt. Finally, add the fenugreek leaves and cover. Leave to cook for further 3 minutes.

## Prawn and Mangetouts Stir Fry    Top Choice ✓    Low Carb

Nutritional Facts: Protein 25g, Carbs 8g, Saturated Fat 0.5g, Unsaturated Fat 3.5g

*Ingredients:*
5 king prawns thawed and peeled or 125-150g of peeled prawns, ¼ tablespoon of oil, ½ a medium onion, ¼ tablespoon of tomato puree, ¼ tsp of tabasco sauce, ¼ tsp of lemon juice, ¼ tsp of ginger pulp, ¼ tsp of garlic pulp, ¼ tsp of chili powder, pinch of salt, ¼ tablespoon of chopped fresh coriander, 4-5 mangetouts halved

*Add to this meal?*
Chapati, Rice, Potato

Heat a little oil in wok or deep frying pan and fry onions over a medium heat until golden brown. Mix the tomato puree with a tablespoon of water and blend the tabasco sauce, lemon juice, chili powder, garlic pulp and touch of salt.

Lower the heat and pour the sauce over the onions, stir frying for 20 seconds, then, add the coriander, prawns and mangetouts and stir fry for 5-6 minutes.

## Monkfish with Vegetables    Top Choice ✓    Low Carb

Nutritional Facts: Protein 30g, Carbs 8g, Saturated Fat 0.4g, Unsaturated Fat 2.5g

*Ingredients:*
150g of Monkfish, ½ tablespoon of oil, ½ medium onion sliced, ¼ tsp garlic pulp, ¼ tsp ground cumin, ¼ tsp ground coriander, ¼ tsp chili powder, ½ tablespoon of fresh fenugreek leaves, 1 tomato seeded and sliced, ½ a courgette sliced, pinch of salt, ¼ tablespoon of lime juice

*Add to this meal?*
Chapati, Rice, Potato

Heat a little oil in wok or deep frying pan and fry onions over a medium heat until golden brown. Then, add in the cumin, garlic, coriander and chili powder and stir fry for a minute. Add the fish and continue to stir fry for 4 minutes. Add the fenugreek, tomatoes, courgette and touch of salt and cook for a further 2 minutes. Sprinkle with lime juice when serving.

## Fish and Vegetable Kebabs  Top Choice ✓  Low Carb

Nutritional Facts: Protein 30g, Carbs 8g, Saturated Fat 0.5g, Unsaturated Fat 3.5g

*Ingredients:*
150g of white fish fillets like cod or haddock, 1 tablespoon of lemon juice, ¼ tsp of ginger pulp, ½ green chili very finely chopped, ¼ tablespoon of very finely chopped fresh coriander, ¼ tablespoon of very finely chopped fresh mint, ¼ tsp of ground coriander, pinch of salt, 1/3 a red or green pepper, ¼ of a medium cauliflower, 3 button mushrooms, 2 cherry tomatoes or half a medium tomato, ¼ tablespoon of oil, ¼ of a lime used to garnish

*Add to this meal?*
Chapati, Rice, Potato

*Preparation:* Cut fish fillets into chunks, then in a mixing bowl mix together the lemon juice, ginger, fresh coriander, chillies, mint, ground coriander and pinch of salt. Add the fish chunks and leave to marinade for 30 minutes. Slice peppers into squares and cut the cauliflower into small florets.

With the grill on maximum, arrange the peppers, cauliflower, mushrooms, tomatoes and fish onto skewers and brush with a little oil. Grill for 7-9 minutes turning occasionally.

## Indian Fish Stew  High Carb

Nutritional Facts: Protein 30g, **Carbs 40g**, Saturated Fat 0.5g, Unsaturated Fat 4.5g

*Ingredients:*
150g of cod fillet, ¼ tablespoon of oil, ¼ tsp of cumin seeds, ¼ of an onion chopped, ¼ of a red pepper seeded and thinly sliced, ¼ of a garlic clove crushed, ½ a red chili finely chopped, ½ a bay leaf, pinch of salt, ¼ tsp of ground cumin, ¼ tsp of ground coriander, ¼ tsp chili powder, 100g of chopped tomatoes, 1 large potato cut into chunks, 50ml of water or fish stock

*Add to this meal?*
Chapatis

Heat a little oil in a wok or deep frying pan and fry the cumin seeds until they begin to splutter. Add the onion, pepper, garlic, chillies and bay leaf and fry for 5 minutes until onions brown. Then, add a pinch of salt, ground cumin and coriander and chili powder and cook for 3 minutes.

Stir in tomatoes, potatoes and water or fish stock, bring to the boil and simmer for 8 minutes. Add the fish and allow to simmer for 10 minutes or until fish and potatoes are tender.

## Cod with Spicy Mushroom Sauce          Low Carb
Nutritional Facts: Protein 25g, Carbs 8g, Saturated Fat 1g, Unsaturated Fat 4g

*Ingredients:*
150g of cod fillet, ¼ tablespoon of lemon juice, ¼ tablespoon of oil, ¼ medium onion chopped, 1 black peppercorn crushed, 40g or 1oz of mushrooms, 45ml of natural low fat yogurt, ¼ tsp of ginger pulp, ¼ tsp of garlic pulp, pinch of garam masala, pinch of chili powder, pinch of salt, ¼ tablespoon of fresh coriander leaves to garnish, served with lightly cooked greena beans

*Add to this meal?*
Chapati, Rice, Potato, Green Beans

*Preparation:* Sprinkle lemon juice on cod fillets then grill for 5 minutes on each side then set aside. Heat a little oil in wok or deep frying pan and fry the onion and peppercorns for a couple of minutes. Lower the heat then add mushrooms and stir fry for 4 minutes.

In a bowl mix the yogurt, garlic and ginger pulp, garam masala, chili and pinch of salt. Pour over the onions and stir fry for 3 minutes. Add the cod fillets to the sauce and cook for a further 2 minutes.

## Spicy Grilled Fish Fillets    Top Choice ✓    Low Carb
Nutritional Facts: Protein 25-30g, Carbs 4g, Saturated Fat 1g, Unsaturated Fat 4g

*Ingredients:*
125-150g (4-5oz) of cod, sole, plaice or flounder, ¼ tsp of garlic pulp, ¼ tsp garam masala, ¼ tsp chili powder, pinch of ground turmeric, pinch of salt, ¼ tablespoon finely chopped fresh coriander, ¼ tablespoon of oil, ½ tablespoon of lemon juice, tomato wedges and grated carrot to ganish

*Add to this meal?*
Chapati, Rice, Potato,

Place foil on an ovenproof dish or pan and place the fish fillets. In a bowl mix the garam masala, garlic, chili powder, turmeric, pinch of salt, lemon juice, oil and coriander. Brush the fillets with the mixture.

Grill the fish for 10 minutes on medium heat. You can add more mixture thorughout if required.

## Tuna Fish Curry — Top Choice ✓ — Low Carb
Nutritional Facts: Protein 30g, Carbs 4g, Saturated Fat 1g, Unsaturated Fat 5.5g

*Ingredients:*
125-150g can of tinned tuna in brine drained, ¼ of an onion, ½ a red or green pepper, ½ tablespoon oil, pinch of cumin seeds, pimch of ground cumin, pinch of ground coriander, pinch of chili powder, pinch of salt, ½ a garlic clove crushed, ¼ green chili finely chopped, ¼ inch of root ginger grated, pinch of garam masala, ¼ of lemon juice, ½ tablespoon of chopped fresh coriander, plus a little to garnish, Pitta breads with Raita to serve

*Add to this meal?*
Wholemeal Pitta Breads

Thinly slice peppers and onion. Heat a little oil in wok or deep frying pan and stir fry the cumin seeds for 2-3 minutes until they begin to splutter. Then, add the cumin, chili powder, coriander and pinch of salt and cook for 2 minutes. Add the garlic, onion and peppers.

Fry the vegetables for 6 minutes until the onion has browned. Stir in the tuna, green chili and ginger and cook for 5 minutes. Then, add the garam masala, lemon and chopped coriander and cook for an additional 3 minutes.

## Masala Steak — High Carb
Nutritional Facts: Protein 30g, Carbs 35g, Saturated Fat 6g, Unsaturated Fat 3.7g

*Ingredients:*
250g of boneless Mutton or Beef from the round portion cut into steaks, 1 medium size onion sliced, 1 large potato, 1 cup of water, Salt to taste, 1 tbsp Oil, ¼ teaspoon ginger paste, ¼ teaspoon garlic paste, ½ teaspoon coriander powder, ¼ teaspoon cumin powder, ¼ teaspoon turmeric powder, pepper to taste

Bake the large potato in tin foil in a pre-heated oven for 1 hour or until soft. Using a large wide pan heat a little oil. Add the onions and fry for 5 minutes. Remove half the quantity of onions and set aside. Add the beef and stir-fry for 10 minutes until the pieces turn brown. Reduce heat to medium and add all the other ingredients except the potato. Mix well. Now, add the pre fried onions and mix well into the steak.

## Keema Curry Lentil Soup   Top Choice ✓   High Carb
Nutritional Facts: Protein 23g, Carbs 34g, Saturated Fat 1.2g, Unsaturated Fat 0.8g

*Ingredients: (4 servings)*
10 oz. ground turkey or chicken (275g), 1 small onion chopped, ½ teaspoon of curry powder, 2 cloves garlic, ½ teaspoon of cumin, ¼ teaspoon ginger, pinch of cinnamon, pinch of cloves, pinch of cayenne pepper, Salt and pepper to taste, 1 carrot shredded, 2 celery sticks, ½ cup of dried lentils, 2 medium potatoes chopped, 4 tablespoons of tomato sauce, 2 cups of chicken broth

First, ground down the turkey, garlic, onion, and all spices (everything down to and including salt and pepper). Then using a heavy based frying pan, gently cook the ingredients. When turkey is no longer pink, add carrots and celery and saute for a few minutes, until they begin to soften. Add all other ingredients and bring to a boil, then simmer for one hour, stirring occasionally, until lentils and potatoes are soft.

## Egg Lentil Curry      Top Choice ✓      High Carb
Nutritional Facts: Protein 17g, Carbs 17g, Saturated Fat 4.0g, Unsaturated Fat 4.0g

*Ingredients: (4 servings)*
75 grams (uncooked) green lentils, 400 ml vegetable stock, 4 eggs (4 whites, 2 yolks), ½ tsp oil, 2 cloves, ¼ tsp black peppercorns, ½ onion (finely diced), ½ tsp red chili flakes (or to taste), ½ tbsp minced garlic, ½ tbsp minced ginger root, ¼ bsp curry powder, 200 gram diced tomatoes (tinned is fine), water, ¼ tsp brown sugar, ¼ tsp garam masala

First, place lentils in heavy based pan with stock and simmer for 15 minutes until soft. Drain and set aside. Meanwhile cook eggs in boiling water for 10 minutes. Drain and allow to cool. Then, heat oil in large saucepan and fry cloves and peppercorns for 2 minutes. Add onion, chili, garlic and ginger and fry for 5-6 minutes. Stir in curry powder and mix through. Remove shells from eggs and cut each in half longways. Stir in tomatoes and brown sugar with water. Simmer for 5 minutes until it thickens. Add eggs, (drained) lentils, and garam masala. Cover and simmer for 5 -10 minutes.

# **Recipes** Vegeterian Dishes

*All meals serve 1 person, simply double ingredients to serve 2.*

*NOTE: The majority of Veg Meals are low protein, therefore it is important to consider adding soy, tofu, lentils, beans to these meals where possible.*
**A cup of cooked lentils/beans (200g) will provide approximately 15-20 grams of protein and 17 grams of carbs, so this is highly suggested with every meal where protein content is below 10g. It is also recommended to supplement with a soy, whey or hemp protein poweder to help meet your daily protein targets.**

*Chili – Use this according to personal taste. Chili will define the strength and heat of your curry.*

## **Low Fat Vegetable Curry**                    Top Choice ✓
Nutritional Facts: Protein 8g, Carbs 12g, Saturated Fat 0.5g, Unsaturated Fat 5g

*Ingredients:*
½ teaspoon of oil, pinch of mustard and cumin seeds, ½ an onion thinly sliced, ½ curry leaf, ½ chopped green chili, ¼ piece of root ginger finely chopped, ¼ tablespoon of curry paste, ½ small cauliflower cut into small florets, ½ a carrot thinly sliced, 30g of french beans sliced, pinch of ground turmeric, pinch of chili powder, pinch of salt, ½ a tomato finely chopped, handful of thawed frozen peas, 40ml of vegetable stock

*Add to this meal?*
Chapati, Rice, Lentils or Beans

**For Meat Eaters** – *Add Prawns or cubes of chicken to this meal (Protein Content 25g)*

Heat the oil in a wok or heavy based saucepan and fry the mustard and cumin seeds until they splutter. Then, add the onion and curry leaf and fry for 4 minutes. Add the chili and ginger and continue to fry for 2 minutes. Stir in the curry paste and fry for a further 2 minutes.

Next, add the cauliflower florets, carrot and beans and continue to cook for 4 minutes. Add the turmeric, chili powder, tomatoes and touch of salt and further cook for 2 minutes. Next, add the peas and cook for 2 minutes. Lastly, add the stock, cover and allow to simmer over a low heat for 10 minutes or until the vegetables are tender.

## Stir Fried Vegetables with Cashews          Top Choice ✓
Nutritional Facts: Protein 10g, Carbs 12g, Saturated Fat 1g, Unsaturated Fat 5.5g

*Ingredients:*
1 medium carrot, 1 medium green or red pepper, 1 courgette, 1 oz green beans, 1-2 spring onions  chopped, touch of oil, 1-2 curry leaves, pinch of cumin seeds, 1 dried red chili, 5-6 cashew nuts, ½ tablespoon of lemon juice, pinch of salt, fresh mint leaves to garnish

*Add to this meal?*
Chappati, Rice, Lentils or Beans

Prepare all the vegetables by washing and then cutting into small pieces or matchsticks. Using a wok or heavy based frying pan, stir fry the curry leaves, dried chillies and cumin seeds for approximately 1 minute. Then, add the vegetables and nuts along with the lemon juice and pinch of salt and continue to fry for 4 minutes. When done garnish with fresh mint leaves.

## Carb Cutting Courgette Curry          Top Choice ✓
Nutritional Facts: Protein 8g, Carbs 15g, Saturated Fat 1g, Unsaturated Fat 6g

*Ingredients:*
160g of courgettes, ¼ tablespoon of oil, ¼ teaspoon of cumin seeds, ¼ teaspoon of mustard seeds, ½ an onion thinly sliced, ½ a garlic clove crushed, pinch of ground turrmeric, pinch of chili powder, pinch of ground coriander, pinch of ground cumin, pinch of salt, ¼ tablespoon of tomato puree, 100g chopped tomatoes, 40ml of water, pinch of garam masala

*Add to this meal?*
Chapati, Rice, Lentils or Beans

Cut the courgettes into thick chunks or slices. Using a wok or heavy based frying plan stir fry the mustard and cumin seeds for 2 minutes until they splutter. Then, add in the onion and garlic and fry for 4 minutes. Next, add the turmeric, chili powder, cumin, ground coriander and pinch of salt and continue frying for 2 minutes.

Add the courgettes and cook for 5 minutes while stirring frequently. Mix in the tomato puree and chopped tomatoes with the water, cover and allow to simmer on low heat for 10 minutes. Stir in fresh coriander and garam masala and continue to cook for 4-5 minutes or until courgettes are cooked.

## Vegetable Kashmiri
Nutritional Facts: Protein 8g, Carbs 30g, Saturated Fat 1g, Unsaturated Fat 7g

*Ingredients:*
½ teaspoon of cumin seeds, 2 black peppercorns, ½ green cardamon pod (seeds only), ½ inch cinnamon stick, pinch of grated nutmeg, ½ tablespoon oil, ¼ green chili, ¼ inch grated root ginger, pinch of chili powder, pinch of salt, ½ a large potato cut into chunks,  2oz of cauliflower cut into florets, 2oz okra trimmed and thickly sliced, 40ml natural low fat yogurt, 40ml vegetable stock, fresh coriander to garnish.

*Add to this meal?*
Chapati, Rice, Soy or Tofu

Taking the cumin seeds, cardamom, peppercorns, cinnamon stick and nutmeg, grind to produce a powder. Small blender or pestle and motor will be useful here.

Heat a little oil in a wok or heavy based frying saucepan and fry the chili powder and ginger for a minute, constantly stirring to avoid sticking. Then add the pinch of salt and spice mixture from earlier and continue frying for 2-3 minutes. Next, add the potatoes, then cover and cook for 10 minutes over a low heat, stirring every two minutes.

Add the cauliflower and okra and cook for an additional 4 minutes. Lastly, add the yogurt and stock. Bring to the boil, then reduce the heat. Cover and allow to simmer for 15-20 miinutes or until vegetables are tender. Garnish with toasted almonds.

## Low Fat Aubergine Curry                                    Top Choice ✓

Nutritional Facts: Protein 8g, Carbs 12g, Saturated Fat 0.5g, Unsaturated Fat 4.5g

*Ingredients:*
1 medium aubergine approx. 100-120g, ¼ tablespoon of oil, pinch of black mustard seeds, 3 spring onions finely chopped, 1oz button mushrooms halved, ½ garlic clove crushed, ¼ red chili finely chopped, pinch of chili powder, pinch of ground cumin, pinch of ground coriander, pinch of ground turmeric, pinch of salt, 100g or 1oz of chopped tomatoes, ¼ tablespoon fresh coriander, fresh coriander to garnish

*Add to this meal?*
Chapati, Rice, Lentils or Beans

Wrap the aubergines in foil and bake in the oven for 1 hour. After cooking, remove from foil and leave to cool down. Next, heat a little oil in heavy based saucepan and fry the mustard seeds for 2 minutes or until they splutter. Then, add the spring onions, garlic, mushrooms and chili and fry for 5 minutes. Stir in the chili powder, ground coriander, cumin, turmeric and pinch of salt and fry for a further 3 minutes. Lastly, add in the tomatoes and allow to simmer on a low heat for 5 minutes.

Then, cut the aubergines in half and scoop out the soft flesh into a bowl. Mash down with a fork. Add the mashed aubergine and fresh coriander to the saucepan. Bring to the boil and simmer for 4 minutes or until sauce thickens up. Serve with sprig or two of fresh coriander.

## Broad Beans and Caulifower Curry

Nutritional Facts: Protein 8g, Carbs 30g, Saturated Fat 0.5g, Unsaturated Fat 7.5g

*Ingredients:*
½ garlic clove chopped. ¼ inch piece of root ginger, ½ fresh green chili seeded and chopped, ¼ tablespoon of oil, ¼ onion sliced, ½ potato chopped, pinch of medium or hot curry powder, ¼ cauliflower cut into florets, 150ml of stock, pinch of salt and black pepper, 2oz of canned broad beans and juice, squeeze of lemon juice (optional), fresh coriander to garnish

*Add to this meal?*
Soy or Tofu for increased protein

Using a blender, blend together the ginger, garlic, chili and oil until a paste forms. In a heavy based saucepan fry the potatoes and onion in a little oil, then stir in the spice paste and curry powder. Cook for 1 minute.

Then, add the cauliflower florets to the saucepan and continue stirring until the mixture is combined, then pour in the stock and bring to the boil. Cover and allow to simmer gently for 10 minutes. Add in the beans and cook uncovered for a further 10 minutes. Lemon juice can be added, along with coriander to garnish.

## Low Carb Masala Beans with Fenugreek
Nutritional Facts: Protein 8g, Carbs 10g, Saturated Fat 0.5g, Unsaturated Fat 4.5g

*Ingredients:*
Pinch of ground cumin, pinch of ground coriander, pinch of sesame seeds, pinch of chili powder, pinch of ground turmeric, pinch of salt, pinch of garlic pulp, ¼ medium onion roughly chopped, hint of oil, small tomato quartered, 2oz green beans, half a bunch of fresh fenugreek leaves (stems disgarded), 1 tablespoon fresh coriander, squeeze of lemon juice

*Add to this meal?*
Rice, Lentils or Beans

Mix together the ground cumin and coriander, chili, turmeric, sesame seeds and pinch of salt. Next, stir in the garlic pulp into the dry spices and add the chopped onion, then place into blender or food processor. Blend into a thick creamy mixture.

Using a heavy based saucepan, heat the oil and fry the spice mixture for 3 minutes. Next, add the green beans, tomatoes, fenugreek and fresh coriander. Stir fry the beans and mixture for 5 minutes. Sprinkle in lemon juice before serving.

## Okra in Yogurt
Nutritional Facts: Protein 8g, Carbs 8g, Saturated Fat 0.4g, Unsaturated Fat 4.5g

*Ingredients:*
100g of okra, hint of oil, pinch of onion seeds, 1 medium green chili chopped, ¼ medium onion sliced, pinch of turmeric, pinch of salt, ½ tablespoon low fat yogurt, 1 small tomato sliced, fresh corainder

*Add to this meal?*
Chapatis, Can be served with Tarka Dhal, see later in this recipe chapter

After washing the okra slice into pieces. Next, heat a little oil in a medium frying pan, add the onion seeds, chillies and onion and fry for 4 minutes until the onion browns. Then, lower the heat, add the turmeric and pinch of salt and fry for a minute.

Add in the okra, increase the heat to medium and stir fry for 5 minutes until they turn golden. Add in the yogurt, tomatoes and coriander and cook for a further 2 minutes.

## Aloo Gobi
Nutritional Facts: Protein 8g, Carbs 25g, Saturated Fat 0.7g, Unsaturated Fat 7.0g

*Ingredients:*
120g of potato or sweet potato cut into chunks, ¼ tablespoon of oil, pinch of cumin seeds, ½ green chili chopped, 120g of cauliflower florets, pinch of ground coriander, pinch of ground cumin, pinch of chili powder, pinch of ground turmeric, pinch of salt, fresh coriander to garnish

Par-boil the potatoes in a saucepan of boiling water for 10 minutes. Drain and set aside until later. Heat a little oil in heavy based frying pan and fry the cumin seeds for 2 minutes until they splutter. Add the chili and fry for an additional minute. Add in the cauliflower and fry for 5 minutes. Lastly add the potatoes and spices along with pinch of salt and cook for a further 8 minutes until vegetables are tender.

## Aloo Saag          Top Choice ✓          High Carb
Nutritional Facts: Protein 8g, Carbs 35g, Saturated Fat 0.5g, Unsaturated Fat 4.5g

*Ingredients:*
120g of spinach, touch of oil, pinch of black mustard seeds, ½ a small onion sliced, ½ garlic clove crushed, ¼ inch piece of root ginger finely chopped, 150g of potato cut into chunks, pinch of chili powder, pinch of salt, 40ml of water

After washing the spinach set aside until later. The spinach needs to be totally dry before using. Using a heavy based saucepan fry the mustard seeds for 2 minutes. Then, add in the onion, garlic clove and ginger and fry for 4 minutes. Next, add in the potato chunks, chili powder, pinch of salt and water and continue to stir fry on medium heat for a further 7 minutes. Add in the dry spinach, cover the pan and allow to simmer for 10-15 minutes until potatoes are cooked.

## Low Fat Okra Masala

Nutritional Facts: Protein 8g, Carbs 10g, Saturated Fat 0.5g, Unsaturated Fat 4.5g

*Ingredients:*
125g of Okra, pinch of ground cumin, pinch of ground coriander, pinch of chili powder, pinch of ground turmeric, pinch of salt, pinch of sugar, squeeze of lemon juice, sprinkle of chopped fresh coriander, touch of oil, pinch of cumin seeds, pinch of mustard seeds, chopped fresh tomatoes to garnish

*Add to this meal?*
Lentils or Beans

Wash the okra and set aside. Using a bowl mix together the chili powder, turmeric, cumin, ground coriander, pinch of salt, pinch of sugar, lemon juice and fresh coriander. Next, heat a little oil in a heavy based frying pan or wok. Add the sumin seeds and mustard seeds and fry until they splutter. Next, add the spice mixture and fry for 2 minutes. Lastly, add in the okra, cover and cook on a low heat for 10 minutes.

## Balti with Sweetcorn and Cauliflower

Nutritional Facts: Protein 8g, Carbs 20g, Saturated Fat 0.5g, Unsaturated Fat 4.0g

*Ingredients:*
Touch of oil, 1 curry leaf, pinch of onion seeds, half a chili seeded and chopped, 2oz of frozen or tinned sweetcorn, ¼ cauliflower cut into florets, 2 mint leaves

*Add to this meal?*
Rice or Bombay Potatoes, Soy or Tofu

Using a wok or heavy based frying pan stir fry the curry leaf and onion seeds for 30 seconds. Add in the onions and fry for five minutes until they turn golden brown. Add the chili, sweetcorn and cauliflower and stir fry for 5 minutes. Lastly, add in the mint leaves and serve.

# Mushrooms and Courgettes in Yogurt

Nutritional Facts: Protein 8g, Carbs 6g, Saturated Fat 0.5g, Unsaturated Fat 4.0g

*Ingredients:*
Touch of oil, ½ small onion chopped, pinch of ground coriander, pinch of ground cumin, pinch of salt, pinch chili powder, 50g of mushrooms sliced, ½ courgette sliced, 1 tablespoon natural low fat yogurt, pinch of fresh coriander

*Add to this meal?*
Rice or Potatoes, Lentils or Beans

Using a wok or heavy based frying pan fry the onions until golden. Then, lower the heat to medium, add in the ground coriander, pinch of salt, cumin and chili powder and stir together. Next, add the mushrooms and courgettes and stir fry gently for 5 minutes. Water can be added if mixture dries up. Lastly, add the yogurt and stir well. Garnish with fresh chopped coriander and serve.

# Kidney Beans with Sweetcorn          Top Choice ✓

Nutritional Facts: Protein 8g, Carbs 6g, Saturated Fat 0.5g, Unsaturated Fat 4.0g

*Ingredients:*
Touch of oil, pinch of mustard seeds, ¼ small red onions, 25g of frozen or tinned sweetcorn, 25g canned red kidney beans, ¼ red chili seeded and diced, ¼ garlic clove chopped, ¼ inch piece of root ginger chopped, pinch of salt, touch of fresh coriander

*Add to this meal?*
Rice or Potatoes, Lentils or Beans

With a wok or heavy based frying pan, add a little oil and heat for 30 seconds, then, stir fry the mustard seeds and onion for 2-3 minutes. Next, add the sweetcorn, red kidney beans and continue to fry for 4 minutes. Then, add the chopped garlic, chili, ginger, coriander and touch of salt and fry for an additional 2-3 minutes. Serve with diced tomato.

## Red Chillies with Potatoes                     High Carb

Nutritional Facts: Protein 8g, Carbs 30g, Saturated Fat 0.5g, Unsaturated Fat 3.5g

*Ingredients:*
4-5 Baby New Potatoes peeled and halved, pinch of salt, touch of oil, pinch of crushed dried red chillies, pinch of cumin seeds, pinch of fennel seeds, pinch of crushed coriander seeds, 1 fresh red chili chopped (for milder version take out the seeds and disgard or use half a chili), pinch of fresh coriander

*Add to this meal?*
Lentils or Beans

Boil the potatoes in a pinch of salt and water until soft and firm or purchase tinned potatoes. Drain water and set aside. In a wok or deep based frying pan, heat a touch of oil, then on a medium heat add the crushed chillies, cumin, coriander, fennel and pinch of salt and stir fry rapidly for 40 seconds. Next, add the onion and fry until golden. Then, add the new potatoes, fresh chillies and fresh coriander. Cover and cook for 6 minutes on a low heat.

## Sweet & Sour Vegetables & Tofu Kebabs

Nutritional Facts: Protein 8g, Carbs 11g, Saturated Fat 0.3g, Unsaturated Fat 3.3g

*Ingredients:*
½ Green Pepper seeded and cut into squares, 4 cherry tomatoes, 4 cauliflower florets, 4 cubes of tofu or panir, 4 pineapple chunks

*Ingredients for Oil:*
Touch of oil, squeeze of lemon juice, pinch of salt, pinch of crushed black peppercorns, pinch of chili sauce, ½ teaspoon of honey

*Add to this meal?*
Rice, Beans or Lentils

Using skewers, thread the green pepper squares, cherry tomatoes, cauliflower florets, pineapple chunks and tofu. Place the skewers under the grill. Using a small bowl mix the ingredients for the oil. Add a little water if this is too thick. Brush the vegetables skewers with the oil and grill for 10 minutes turning from time to time.

# Vegetables, Beans and Curry Leaves
Nutritional Facts: Protein 8g, Carbs 15g, Saturated Fat 0.3g, Unsaturated Fat 3.3g

*Ingredients:*
Touch of oil, 1-2 curry leaves, 1 garlic clove sliced, 1 dried red chili, pinch of onion seeds, pinch of fenugreek seeds, 1 fresh green chili chopped, 40g or 1oz of canned red kidney beans, ½ medium carrot cut into strips, 1 green bean sliced, ½ medium red pepper seeded and cut into strips, pinch of salt, squeeze of lemon juice.

*Add to this meal?*
Rice

Using a wok or heavy based frying pan heat a touch of oil and add in the curry leaves, garlic clove, dried chillies and onion/fenugreek seeds. Fry until the ingredients begin to darken, then, add the chillies, kidney beans, carrots, green beans sliced and pepper strips. Add a pinch of salt and lemon juice. Lower the heat, cover and cook for an additional 5 minutes.

# Sweetcorn and Pea Curry        High Carb
Nutritional Facts: Protein 8g, Carbs 30g, Saturated Fat 0.5g, Unsaturated Fat 5.0g

*Ingredients:*
1 corn on the cob cut into three or four chunks, touch of oil, pinch of cumin seeds, ½ small onion finely chopped, ½ garlic clove crushed, ½ green chili finely chopped, 5ml curry paste, pinch of ground coriander, pinch of ground cumin, pinch of ground turmeric, pinch of salt, pinch of sugar, 100g or 4oz chopped tomatoes, touch of tomato puree, 40ml of water, 40g of peas, fresh coriander

*Add to this meal?*
Rice, Beans or Lentils

Taking the corn on the cob, cut into 6 smaller chunks. Bringing a large pan of water to the boil, add the corns and cook for 10-12 minutes, then drain. Next, heat a little oil in a heavy based saucepan and fry the cumin seeds for 2 minutes. Add the onion, garlic and chili and fry for 5-6 minutes.

Then, add the curry paste and fry for a further 1 minute. Stir in the remaining spices, pinch of salt and sugar and fry for a further 2-3 minutes, adding a little water if mixture gets too dry. Add the chopped tomatoes and puree together with the water and simmer for 5 minutes or until the mixture begins to thicken.

Then, add the peas and cook for a further 4 minutes. Add the corns and fresh coriander and cook for a final 7 minutes.

## Vegetables with Almonds
Nutritional Facts: Protein 8g, Carbs 10g, Saturated Fat 1.3g, Unsaturated Fat 10g

*Ingredients:*
Touch of oil, ½ small onion sliced, ½ inch of root ginger shredded, pinch of crushed black peppercorns, pinch of ground turmeric, pinch of ground coriander, pinch of salt, 45g of mushrroms thickly sliced, ½ medium courgette thickly sliced, pinch of chopped fresh mint, 40ml of water, 1 tablespoon of natural low fat yogurt, flaked almonds to garnish

*Add to this meal?*
Rice, Beans or Lentils

Heat a touch of oil in a wok or heavy based frying pan and fry the onions until golden. Also mix in the ginger, peppercorns and bay leaf add fry for a further 3-4 minutes. Lower the heat and add in the turmeric, ground coriander, pinch of salt and garam masala, stirring occasionally. Gradually add the sliced mushrooms, courgette, mint and green beans.

Pour in water and bring to a simmer, then lower the heat and cook until the water has been totally absorbed by the vegetables. Pour in the yogurt and mix together until everything is coated. Cook for a further 2-3 minutes. Garnish with flaked almonds.

## Stir Fry with Cauliflower and Carrot          Top Choice ✓
Nutritional Facts: Protein 8g, Carbs 10g, Saturated Fat 0.5g, Unsaturated Fat 3.7g

*Ingredients:*
1 medium carrot, ¼ small cauliflower cut into florets, touch of oil, ¼ small cinnamon stick, ½ cardamom pod, touch of black pepper, pinch of salt, 1oz or 25g of peas, ¼ tablespoon of lemon juice, pinch of fresh coriander and some to garnish

*Add to this meal?*
Rice, Potatoes, Beans or Lentils
Cut the carrots into thin slices and cut the cauliflower into small florets. Using a

wok or heavy based pan, heat a little oil and add the bay leaf, cinnamon stick, cardamom pod and touch of black pepper. Over a medium heat fry for 30 seconds, then add the pinch of salt. Next, add the sliced carrot and cauliflower and continue to fry for 4 minutes. Finally, add the peas, lemon juice and coriander and cook for a further 4 minutes.

## Balti Potatoes with Aubergines — High Carb

Nutritional Facts: Protein 8g, Carbs 35g, Saturated Fat 0.7g, Unsaturated Fat 4.0g

*Ingredients:*
4-5 Baby Potatoes, 1-2 Small Aubergines, ¼ red pepper, touch of oil, ½ mediun onion sliced, 1-2 curry leaves, pinch of onion seeds, pinch of crushed coriander seeds, pinch of cumin seeds, ¼ teaspoon of ginger pulp, ¼ teaspoon of garlic pulp, pinch of crushed dried red chillies, ¼ tablespoon chopped fresh fenugreek, pinch of chopped fresh coriander, ¼ tablespoon natural low fat yogurt, fresh coriander leaves to garnish

Tip: Choose small aubergines if possible as they contain more flavor

First cook the potatoes (unpeeled) in a large saucepan of boiling water. Don't let them break down, they should remain soft. Then, set them aside. With the aubergines, cut them into smaller pieces, also cut the pepper and remove the seeds, then cut into strips. Using a wok or heavy baseed frying pan heat a little oil and add in the sliced onions, onions seeds, curry leaves, coriander seeds and cumin seeds. Fry until the onion begins to golden.

Next, add the ginger, garlic, fenugreek, chillies and aubergines and stir fry together. Cover and allow to cook on a low heat for 6 minutes. Lastly, add a litle fresh coriander before serving.

## Baked Potato with Spicy Cottage Cheese — High Carb

Nutritional Facts: Protein 12g, Carbs 25g, Saturated Fat 0.5g, Unsaturated Fat 4.3g

*Ingredients:*
1 medium baking potato, 75g of low fat cottage cheese, ½ teaspoon of tomato puree, pinch of ground cumin, pinch of ground coriander, pinch of chili powder, touch of oil, pinch of onion and mustard seeds, 1 curry leaf, 10ml of water

*For Garnish:*

mixed salad leaves, fresh coriander

First wrap the potato in foil and bake for one hour at 180 degrees. Next, in a mixing bowl add the tomato puree, cumin, coriander and chili powder and mix together.

In a saucepan, heat some oil and then add in the mustard and onion seeds and the curry leaves, give a few tilts to let the oil soak the ingredients. After approximtely 45 seconds pour in the mixture from the bowl and place on low heat. Add the water and mix. Place 75g of low fat cottage cheese in a bowl (add more if you want to increase protein content) and then pour the mixture over the cheese and mix together.

Once the potato is cooked to your liking, cut through with a knife and pour the cottage cheese mixture into the potato.

## Yogurt Covered Potatoes      High Carb
Nutritional Facts: Protein 10g, Carbs 28g, Saturated Fat 0.8g, Unsaturated Fat 4.3g

*Ingredients:*
1 medium baked potato chunked, 70g low fat natural yogurt, 75ml of water, pinch of ground turmeric, pinch of chili powder, pinch of ground coriander, pinch of ground cumin, pinch of salt, touch of oil, pinch of cumin seeds, pinch of chopped fresh coriander

Boil the potato chunks in the skin until tender, drain and set aside for later. For the yogurt sauce, mix together the yogurt, turmeric, chili powder, water, ground coriander, cumin and pinch of salt. Set this aside.

Using a heavy based saucepan, heat a touch of oil and then fry the cumin seeds for 1 minute. Then, reduce the heat and add in the yogurt mixture and cook for 3 minutes. Lastly, add the chopped fresh coriander, green chillies and potato chunks. Mix it all together and cook for an additional 6 minutes.

# Kidney Bean Curry                                    High Carb

Nutritional Facts: Protein 18g, Carbs 35g, Saturated Fat 0.8g, Unsaturated Fat 7.0g

*Ingredients:*
60g tinned red kidney beans, ½ tablespoon of oil, pinch of cumin seeds, ¼ onion thinly sliced, ½ green chili finely chopped, ½ a garlic clove crushed, ½ tablespoon of curry paste, pinch of ground cumin, pinch of ground coriander, pinch of chili powder, pinch of salt, 100g of chopped tomatoes, fresh coriander to garnish

First drain the tinned beans and set aside as these are already cooked. Then, using a wok or heavy based frying pan, heat a little oil and fry the cumin seeds for 2 minutes. Then, add in the onion, garlic, ginger and chili and stir fry for 3 minutes. Next, stir in the curry paste, ground coriander, cumin, chili powder and pinch of salt and cook for an additional 4 minutes.

Add in the tomatoes and simmer for 4 minutes. Then, add the kidney beans, cover and cook on low heat for 10 minutes. Add a little coriander to garnish.

# Tarka Dhal

Nutritional Facts: Protein 8g, Carbs 20g, Saturated Fat 0.8g, Unsaturated Fat 6.0g

*Ingredients:*
40g or 1oz of red split lentils, 150ml of water, ¼ teaspoon of ginger pulp, ¼ teaspoon of garlic pulp, pinch of ground turmeric, ½ green chili chopped, pinch of salt

*For the Tarka:*
½ tablespoon of oil, ½ a small onion sliced, pinch of mixed mustard and onion seeds, 1 dried red chili, ½ a tomato sliced

*For the Garnish:*
Pinch of chopped fresh coriander, ½ a fresh green chili seeded and sliced, pinch of chopped fresh mint

Boil the lentils in water with garlic and ginger pulp, chopped green chillies and turmeric for 15 minutes. If not soft cook for a little longer. Then, mash the mixture with a utensil until the consistency changes to a thick soup. You can add a little more water if required.

Season with a pinch of salt. For the Tarka, using a wok or heavy based frying pan, heat a little oil and add in the onion and mustard seeds, dried chillies and tomato and fry for 1-2 minutes. Pour the Tarka over the lentils. Garnish with a little fresh coriander.

## Spinach Dhal                              Top Choice ✓
Nutritional Facts: Protein 8g, Carbs 20g, Saturated Fat 0.4g, Unsaturated Fat 2.0g

*Ingredients:*
45g of yellow split peas, 45ml of water, touch of oil, pinch of black mustard seeds, ½ an onion thinly sliced, ½ garlic clove crushed, ¼ inch piece of root ginger grated or pinch of ground ginger, ¼ red chili finely chopped, 80g of canned or frozen spinach, pinch of chili powder, pinch of ground coriander, pinch of garam masala, pinch of salt

Wash the yellow plit peas and then allow to soak in water for 30 minutes. Then, drain the yellow split peas and place in a heavy based saucepan with water and bring to the boil, cover and allow to simmer for 20-25 minutes.

Using a wok or heavy based frying pan, heat a touch of oil and fry the mustard seeds until they splutter. Next, add in the onion, ginger, garlic and chili and fry for 5 minutes. Add the spinach and cook for 8 minutes or until the spinach is dry. Stir in all the remaining spices and cook for a further 1-2 minutes. Drain the peas and add to the pan. Cook for a further 4 minutes.

## Spinach and Lentil Soup              Top Choice ✓
Nutritional Facts: Protein 6g, Carbs 16g, Saturated Fat 1.0g, Unsaturated Fat 2.2g

*Ingredients:*
Olive Oil ½ tbsp, Garlic 1 clove chopped finely, ½ an onion chopped, pepper powder, paprika and cayenne, pinch of all, Coriander powder ½ tsp, Split red Lentils ½ cup, Red RipeTomatoes ½ cup - chopped or sliced, Spinach frozen 5oz, Ginger Root ½ tsp grated, Cilantro 1 tbsp

Heat a heavy based saucepan, add olive oil. When it is heated, add chopped garlic, stir and brown. Add chopped onion, stir and cook until transparent. Add all the powders, brown for 30 seconds, stir in washed split lentils with 2 cups of water. Cook on hot until the mixture starts boiling. Lower the heat one level, cover tight and cook for 10 minutes or until the lentils are soft. Add 2 more cups of water, chopped tomatoes, defrosted spinach and salt. Cook another 10 minutes until lentils are tender, spinach is cooked and the soup is nice and thick. Garnish with shredded ginger and fresh chopped cilantro leaves. Makes 2 servings.

## Upma                                                    High Carb
Nutritional Facts per Upma: Protein 4g, Carbs 25g, Saturated Fat 1.0g, Unsaturated Fat 3.0g

*Ingredients:*
Olive Oil, 1 tbsp or Ghee, Yellow Mustard seed 1 tsp, Split black gram (Urad dal), 1 tsp, 1 red ot chili cut in half, Fresh green chili Peppers, 1 pepper split in half, Cream of Wheat Cereal (Farina, Soji), 1 cup, 1 cup of hot water (8 fl oz), 1 teaspoon of salt, 2 teaspoon of ginger root (optional)
Fresh curry leaf, 5 leaves ripped in halves.

Heat clarified butter in a deep based saucepan or wok with a tight cover, then drop in mustard seeds. As they start to splutter, add split black gram, red chili, followed by curry leaves and green chili split in half. Stir and add cream of wheat, fry till fragrant for approximately 3 minutes, without letting go of the spoon. Then, stir in the fine chopped ginger. Add salt to water and stir until it's disintegrated. Pour quickly over the farina/soji and mix well. Cover tight and let cook on low heat for about 3 minutes or less, stirring once. It will be dry and crumbly.

Another taste option is to stir in peanuts, cashews, raisins or almonds before adding farina.

## Upma Style Oats                                         High Carb
Nutritional Facts: Protein 7.5g, Carbs 34g, Saturated Fat 3.0g, Unsaturated Fat 4.2g

*Ingredients:*
Steel Cut Oats 40g or half a cup, Clarified butter/Ghee ½ tbsp, Yellow Mustard seed ½ tbsp, Split Black Gram (Urad Dal) ½ tsp, *Hot Chili Peppers ½ tsp pepper chopped fine, 2 slices of Ginger Root shredded, Pinch of salt, Granulated Sugar ½ tsp, 5 fresh curry leaves cut in half, 1 tsp of shredded coconut for garnish.

You can add nuts, raisins, etc. also as an option for variety.

This is prepared exactly the same as Upma. You can make upma also using split mung beans (cook only till mung is tender - yum), grits, Quaker whole oats, vermicelli, etc. for a light breakfast.

## Mattar Panir with Chives

Nutritional Facts: Protein 9.0g, Carbs 11g, Saturated Fat 3.0g, Unsaturated Fat 4.2g

*Ingredients:*
4 oz of frozen peas, 2 oz of fresh panir, 1 teaspoon of olive oil, 1 small onion chopped, ¼ ginger root peeled and shredded, Pinch of cumin powder or seeds, Pinch of coriander powder or seeds, Pinch of cayenne pepper, ¼ sprig of fresh cilantro, Pinch of turmeric, 2 tbsp of Philidelphia Chives and Onion Cream Cheese, 1 small tomato slices, diced and crushed

In a medium sauce pan or heavy base frying pan, heat olive oil and add in the onions and fry until golden. Add the rest of the onions and all the spice powders and fry until brown. Add the shredded ginger and fry again for 30 seconds. Then, add the cream cheese and let the heat melt while you mix it throughly without letting the spoon go to not burn. Stir in the frozen peas, crushed tomatoes, a cup of water and turmeric powder. Mix well, add salt to taste, cover and let come to a boil. Reduce heat to simmer. Add the frozen panir and let cook on a low heat until all the spices are absorbed by the peas and panir. When tender and done, add the cilantro to garnish.

## Maida and Urad Dosa

Nutritional Facts per dosa: Protein 5.0g, Carbs 18g, Saturated Fat 1.2g, Unsaturated Fat 1.0g

*Ingredients: (Makes 5-6 Dosas)*
1/2 cup of Split black gram (Urad Dal), 1 cup of wholegrain flour, pinch or two of salt, 2 teaspoon of oil - 1/2 tsp per dosa or use Pam Spray if available or grape seed oil spray.

First, soak the Urad dal for 4 hours until soft. Then, rinse, drain and blend in a blender until smooth. Let it sit overnight in a warm, dry and dark place. Next, pour water over the wholewheat flour to fully immerse in water and let stand overnight. In the morning, throw away the clear water on top and use the rest to mix well with salt and Urad dal paste to make a batter.

Pour 1/2 a cup on a hot pan smeared with olive oil or spray and spread like you would a french crepe, cover and cook. Remove cover in 20 seconds, turn over after 5 seconds. Brown the other side and serve hot with chutney.

- Tofu can be added to increase protein content.

## Red Lentil Dhal

Nutritional Facts per serving: Protein 14g, Carbs 21g, Saturated Fat 1.4g, Unsaturated Fat 2.6g

*Ingredients: (serves 4-5)*
3 tablespoons peanut oil, 1 medium yellow onion, 1 tablespoon fresh ginger grated, 4 garlic cloves minced, 1 teaspoon salt, 1 cup dried red lentils, 2 tablespoon tomato paste, 4-5 cups veg broth, 5 plum tomatoes chopped, Juice of 1 lime, 1 cup lightly packed chopped fresh cilantro

*Ingredients for Spice Blend:*
2 teaspoons of mustard seeds, 1 teaspoon fenugreek seeds, 1 teaspoon coriander seeds, 1 teaspoon cumin seeds, 6 whole cloves, 4 cardomom pods, 2 dried red chilis (seeds removed), ¼ teaspoon ground cinnamon

In a deep based frying pan or wok over medium heat, toast the seeds (but not the dried red chili) for about 5 minutes, stirring frequently. Remove from pan and let cool. Transfer to coffee grinder, along with the dried red chili and cinnamon, and grind to a fine powder.

Over medium-high heat oil in a soup pot, add onions and fry for 5 minutes. Add garlic and ginger and fry for a further 5 more minutes. Add spices and salt, and fry for an additional 4 minutes more. Then, add 4 cups of water and stir to deglaze the pot. Add tomato paste and lentils. Bring to a boil then lower the heat a bit and simmer for 20 minutes. Add the tomatoes, lime juice and cilantro and more water if it looks to thick. Simmer 10 more minutes, or until lentils are completely tender.

## Scrambled Tofu

Nutritional Facts per serving: Protein 25g, Carbs 19g, **Saturated Fat 24g, Unsaturated Fat 21g**

*Ingredients: (serves 1-2)*
½ yellow onion diced, ½ green bell pepper diced, 1 block tofu drained and pressed, 2 tbsp oil or margarine, 1 tsp garlic powder, 1 tsp onion powder, 1 tbsp light soy sauce, 2 tbsp yeast, ½ tsp turmeric (optional)

Slice the tofu into approximately one inch cubes. Then, using either your hands or a fork, crumble it slightly. Fry onion, pepper and crumbled tofu in oil for 3-5 minutes, stirring often. Add remaining ingredients, reduce heat to medium and allow to cook 5-7 more minutes, stirring frequently and adding more oil if needed.

Wrap in a warmed wholewheat tortilla or Chapati with a spoonful of salsa for a breakfast burrito.

## Tofu and Vegetable Stir Fry with Ginger

Nutritional Facts per serving: Protein 25g, Carbs 20g, **Saturated Fat 24g, Unsaturated Fat 21g**

*Ingredients: (serves 1-2)*
¾ cup soy sauce, ½ cup lemon juice, 1 tbsp fresh ginger, grated or minced, 1 block firm or extra-firm tofu well pressed and cut into 1 inch cubes, 2 tbsp vegetable or olive oil, 1/2 cauliflower, chopped, 1 bunch broccoli chopped, 2 carrots sliced, 1 onion, chopped, 1 bell pepper sliced, 1 cup snow peas, 1 cup mushrooms sliced, 3 green onions (scallions) sliced

In a large shallow bowl, whisk together the soy sauce, lemon juice and ginger. Marinade the tofu in this sauce for at least one hour. In a wok or a large skillet, cook the cauliflower, broccoli, carrots, onion, bell pepper and tofu over high heat, stirring frequently. Add the snow peas, mushrooms, green onions and marinade from the tofu. Allow to cook for just a few more minutes. Vegetables should be tender but not soft.

*Serve with rice, lentils or wholegrains*

# **Recipes** Sides & Salads

*All meals serve 1 person, simply double ingredients to serve 2.*

## Sweet and Sour Raita                          Top Choice ✓
Nutritional Facts: Protein 9g, Carbs 10g, Saturated Fat 0.3g, Unsaturated Fat 1.0g

*Ingredients:*
125ml of natural low fat yogurt, pinch of salt, pinch of sugar, ½ a tablespoon of honey, ½ a teaspoon of mint sauce, two sprinkles of fresh chopped coriander, ¼ green chili seeded and finely chopped, ¼ of a medium onion diced, 15ml of water

Pour yogurt into mxing bowl and add in the pinch of salt, honey, and mint sauce. Add a little of the coriander to the mixture along with the chili, onion and water. Whisk together and pour into serving bowl. Garnish with remainder of fresh coriander.

* Raitas are a great accompanyment to most Indian Meals.

## Sweet Potato and Carrot Salad              Top Choice ✓
Nutritional Facts: Protein 13g, Carbs 25g, Saturated Fat 0.5g, Unsaturated Fat 3.5g

*Ingredients:*
½ a medium sweet potato, ½ a carrot cut into diagonal slices, 1 small tomato, 2-3 lettuce leaves, 20g of tinned chick-peas drained

*Dressing:*
¼ teaspoon clear honey, 25ml of natural low fat yogurt, pinch of salt, pinch of ground black pepper

*For the Garnish:*
Pinch of walnuts, pinch of sultanas,

Peel and wash sweet potato and roughly dice. Boil until soft, remove from heat and set aside to cool. Boil the carrots for approximately 5 minutes, ensuring they remain crunchy. Add the carrots to sweet potatoes, drain and place together in bowl. Chop the tomato and mix together the lettuce, sweet potatoes, carrots, chick peas and tomatoes. Blend the dessing ingredients with a fork. Garnish the salad and then add the walnuts and pinch of sultanas.

## Spinach and Mushroom Salad                    Top Choice ✓
Nutritional Facts: Protein 10g, Carbs 5g, Saturated Fat 0.9g, Unsaturated Fat 0.6g

*Ingredients:*
3 Baby Corn Cobs, 30g of mushrooms, ½ a medium tomato, 5 spinch leaves, 3 onion rings, salad cress (optional), pinch of salt and pepper, fresh coriander to garnish

Slice the corn cobs, mushrooms and tomatoes, Arrange all salad ingredients into a bowl, season with pinch of salt, pepper and garnish with fresh coriander.

## Yogurt Salad                    Top Choice ✓
Nutritional Facts: Protein 10g, Carbs 23g, Saturated Fat 0.9g, Unsaturated Fat 0.4g

*Ingredients:*
90ml of natural low fat yogurt, ¼ teaspoon of clear honey, ½ medium carrot sliced, 1 spring onion chopped, 40g of finely chopped cabbage, 10-15g of sultanas, 4 grapes halved, pinch of salt, fresh mint to garnish

Mix together the yogurt and honey with a fork. Then, mix together the carrots, spring onions, cabbage, sultanas, grapes, pinch of salt and chopped mint. Pour yogurt mixture over the salad and blend together with fork.

## Spicy Vegetable Baby Salad
Nutritional Facts: Protein 8g, Carbs 10g, Saturated Fat 0.4g, Unsaturated Fat 3.1g

*Ingredients:*
3 Baby New Potatoes, 4 Baby Carrots, 3 Baby Courgettes, 30g of button mushrooms,

*For Dressing:*
1 Tablespoon Lemon Juice, ½ tablespoon of oil, pinch of fresh coriander, pinch

of salt, ½ small green chili finely sliced

Boil potatoes, courgettes and carrots until tender. When drained place them with mushrooms. In a different bowl mix all the dressing ingredients. Toss everything together and serve.

## Healthy Salad in Garlic Dressing        Top Choice ✓
Nutritional Facts: Protein 6g, Carbs 10g, Saturated Fat 0.5g, Unsaturated Fat 1.0g

*Ingredients:*
5 Spinach Leaves, 5 Lettuce leaves, ¼ red pepper, 1 medium tomato, 1-2 large tinned pineapple slice, 2 garlic cloves, splash of malt vinegar, touch of oil, pinch of mustard paste, pinch of black pepper

After washing the spinach and lettuce leaves tear them roughly. Roast the red pepper in oven after lightly brushing with oil. Once blistered, peel the skin off and halve the pepper. Deseed and cut into strips. Halve the tomato and cut into small strips or quarters. Cut pineapple slice into strips. Blanch baby corns in hot water for 10 minutes if not already tender. Peel and chop garlic, combine the malt vinegar, oilve oil, garlic, mustard paste and pepper to produce the dressing. Then, place the red peppers, corns, tomatoes and pineapple in dish and gently mix in the lettuce and spinach. Finally, dress with the mixture.

## Leafy Greens with Apple Vinaigrette
Nutritional Facts: Protein 3g, Carbs 12g, Saturated Fat 1.5g, Unsaturated Fat 2.5g

*Ingredients:*
5 Lettuce leaves, 5 spinach leaves, 5 radish leaves,

*Dressing:*
2-3 tablespoons of apple juice, touch of oil, 1 tablespoon red wine vinegar, pinch of paprika, ¼ teaspoon of honey, pinch of black pepper, pinch of salt

Mix all the dressing ingredients in a bottle or shaker and refrigerate until you require. Wash the cabbage and slice into one inch sized pieces. After washing the greens (lettuce etc.) tear into bite size pieces, mix well. To serve add the dressing and toss.

## Red Kidney Bean Salad                    Top Choice ✓

Nutritional Facts: Protein 7g, Carbs 15g, Saturated Fat 0.2g, Unsaturated Fat 0.5g

*Ingredients:*
125g of tinned red kidney beans, ½ a small onion, 1 tablespoon of fresh coriander, pinch of mint, ½ a green chili, 1 tablespoon of lemon juice, ½ teaspoon of chaat masala

Boil the beans, drain and let cool. Peel and cut onion into slices. Add together with the mint and coriander along with the finely sliced chili. Stir in the lemon juice and chaat masala. Refrigerate the dressing for an hour. When cooled, mix in the beans with diced onion and add the dressing. Toss the salad.

## Lassi

Nutritional Facts: Protein 8g, Carbs 8g, Saturated Fat 0.6g, Unsaturated Fat 2.6g

*Ingredients:*
80ml of natural low fat yogurt, pinch of sugar or sweetener, 80ml of water, 1 teaspoon of pureed fruit (optional), pinch of crushed pistachio nuts to garnish

Using a jug or mixing bowl whisk the yogurt until frothy, then add sweetener or pinch of sugar. Pour in the water and pureed fruit (optional) and whisk for 2 minutes. Pour the lassi into a glass and serve.

## Baida Roti

Nutritional Facts: Protein 17g, Carbs 15g, Saturated Fat 3.0g, Unsaturated Fat 2.5g

*Ingredients:*
½ cup of refined white or wholewheat flour, 1 egg, 1 teaspoon of oil, pinch of baking soda,

*Filling Ingredients:*
4 egg whites, touch of oil, 1 small onion chopped, 25g of minced mutton, 1 green chili, pinch of salt, pinch of garam masala, pinch of fresh coriander

Mix together the refined flour, baking powder and egg. Add 2 tablespoons of water and knead into a soft dough and shape into a ball. Cover with a damp cloth and set aside as you prepare the filling.

Heat one teaspoon of oil in a hot frying pan, add the onion and fry until golden. Then, add the minced mutton, green chillies and pinch of salt and cook over medium heat until the mince is cooked and dry. Add thre garam masala and coriander and mix.

Beat four egg whites in a bowl and set aside. Next, roll the dough ball into an 8 inch square chappati. Heat a non stick pan and place the chappati on it. Place some of the mince mixture in the center and add two tablespoons of beaten egg over it. Fold in the sides to make a square package. Pour the rest of the beaten egg over the roti so it sticks to the square and is covered in egg on all sides. Gently continue to fry until crisp. Ad a little chopped onion and fresh coriander to garnish.

## Masala Mashed Potato                                 Side Dish
Nutritional Facts: Protein 5g, Carbs 17.5g, Saturated Fat 1.0g, Unsaturated Fat 5.0g

*Ingredients:*
1 medium potato, pinch of chopped fresh mint and coriander, pinch of mango powder, pinch of salt, pinch of black peppercorns, ½ red chili chopped, 1 tablespoon of low fat margarine

Boil the potatoes and then mash down. Blend all the other ingredients in a bowl. Stir the spice mixture onto the mashed potatoes. Mix together with a fork and serve warm.

## Balti Potatoes                                        Side Dish
Nutritional Facts: Protein 5g, Carbs 17g, Saturated Fat 0.3g, Unsaturated Fat 5.0g

*Ingredients:*
Touch of oil, pinch of cumin seeds, 1 curry leaf, pinch of crushed dried red chillies, pinch of mixed onion/mustard and fenugreek seeds, pinch of fennel seeds, 1 garlic clove sliced, ¼ inch piece of root ginger grated, ½ a medium onion sliced, 3-4 new potatoes or half a large potato chunked, pinch of chopped fresh coriander, ½ a red chili seeded and sliced, ½ red pepper

Cook the potatoes or large potato in a saucepan of boiling water until soft or buy tinned new potatoes and then drain. Cut the half a red pepper into slices. Heat a little oil in a wok or heavy based frying pan and fry the sliced onion, curry leaf, onions seeds, cumin seeds and fennel seeds, stirring frequently. Then, add the ginger, garlic clove, crushed chillies, fenugreek and potatoes. Stir everything together and cover. Lower the heat and cook for 7 minutes. Lastly, remove the lid, add fresh coriander.

## Chapati Masala Noodles 100 Calories Side Dish

Nutritional Facts: Protein 5g, Carbs 17g, Saturated Fat 0.3g, Unsaturated Fat 5.0g

*Ingredients:*
½ tsp low-fat butter, 1/8 cup sliced onions, 1/8 cup sliced capsicum, ¼ piece finely chopped garlic, 1/8 cup tomato slices, 1/8 tsp turmeric powder, 1/8 tsp chili powder, 1/8 tsp black salt (sanchal), 1/8 tsp kitchen king masala, salt to taste, 1 ¼ leftover chapatis cut into long strips

*For The Garnish*
½ tbsp chopped coriander (dhania), lemon wedges to serve

Heat the butter in a heavy based frying pan, add the onions and capsicum and sauté on a medium flame till the onions turn golden. Sprinkle a little water to avoid the onions and capsicum from burning. Then, add the garlic, tomatoes, turmeric powder and chili powder and sauté on a medium flame for another 5 minutes.

Add the black salt, kitchen king masala and salt and mix well. Add the chapati strips and toss well. Serve hot garnished with coriander and lemon wedges!

## Chickpea Patties Side Dish

Nutritional Facts: Protein 7g, Carbs 11g, Saturated Fat 0.5g, Unsaturated Fat 2.0g

*Ingredients:*
1 cup of white chickpeas soaked in water for 8 hours, 1 peeled potato, 2 slices of wholewheat bread, Chopped Coriander leaves, pinch of salt, ¼ tsp turmeric powder, ¼ tsp coriander powder, ¾ tsp garam masala, 1 tsp kitchen king masala, pinch of chili powder

Pressure cook chickpea and potato together until soft. Set aside to cool. Drain the water and add spice powders, coriander leaves and pinch of salt. Them, dry grind bread slices coarsely and add half of it to the chickpea mixture and spread the rest on a plate.

Mash the mixture well. Form balls, flatten, coat both sides with the bread crumbs. Using a wok or deep based frying plan heat 1 tsp of oil. Place patties, drizzle a few drops of oil around the corners and shallow fry on one side for about 3-4 minutes or til golden brown on low flame. Flip them over, drizzle a little more oil and fry till golden brown for 3 minutes. Nice with a little ketchup!

## Brown Idli                                    Side Dish
Nutritional Facts: Protein 2g, Carbs 14g, Saturated Fat 0.5g, Unsaturated Fat 2.0g

*Ingredients:*
2 cups brown rice, 1 cup Urad Daal (white), ½ tblsp Salt, a pinch of Baking Soda, oil for greasing

**Note:** 24 hours preparation time is required for this recipe

Pick, wash and soak the daal overnight. Pick, wash and drain the rice. Grind it coarsely in a blender. Then, grind the daal into a smooth and frothy paste. Next, mix the grinded rice and daal together into a batter. Mix salt and set aside in a warm place for 8-9 hours or overnight for fermenting. Idlis are ready to be cooked when the batter is well fermented. Grease the idli holder or pan well and fill each of them with batter. Steam cook idlis on medium flame for about 10 minutes or until done. Use a knife to remove the idlis. Serve them with sambhar or chutney.

## Wholemeal Chapati                             Side Dish
Nutritional Facts Per Chappati: Protein 2g, Carbs 10g, Saturated Fat 0.5g, Unsaturated Fat 2.0g

*Ingredients to make 10-12 Chapatis:*
350g or 3 cups of wholemeal flour, 2 pinches of salt, water, a little oil for brushing

First, sift the flour and salt into a large mixing bowl, slowly adding small quantities of water until you have a smooth dough. Knead the dough. Then divide it into 10-12 equal portions using one portion at a time and keeping the rest covered. Knead each portion into a ball, then flatten out with your hands and place over flour. Roll out the dough until you have a circle about 7-8".

Heat a griddle and once hot cook one chapati at a time pressing the edges firmly down until both sides are cooked. A little oil can be brushed.

## Maida and Urad Dosa
Nutritional Facts: Protein 5.0g, Carbs 18g, Saturated Fat 1.2g, Unsaturated Fat 1.0g

*Ingredients: (Makes 5-6 Dosas)*
1/2 cup of Split black gram (Urad Dal), 1 cup of wholegrain flour, pinch or two of salt, 2 teaspoon of oil - 1/2 tsp per dosa or use Pam Spray if available or grape seed oil spray

First, soak the Urad dal for 4 hours until soft. Then, rinse, drain and blend in a blender until smooth. Let it sit overnight in a warm, dry and dark place. Next, pour water over the wholewheat flour to fully immerse in water and let stand overnight. In the morning, throw away the clear water on top and use the rest to mix well with salt and Urad dal paste to make a batter.

Pour ½ a cup on a hot pan smeared with olive oil or spray and spread likeyou would a french crepe, cover and cook. Remove cover in 20 seconds, turn over after 5 seconds. Brown the other side and serve hot with chutney.

# **Low Fat** Rices

**One thing that will need to change with your diet is the elimination of White Rice.** If you want that rock hard body white rice has to go and instead be replaced with **Brown or Basmati Rice.** These rices are considered low GI and are much healthier and better in terms of nutrition. You can buy rice in store or prepare your own variations.

All rice recipes below serve 1-2 people.

## Vegetable Pilau Rice                                    High Carb
Nutritional Facts:  Carbs 40g, Saturated Fat 0.5g, Unsaturated Fat 2.5g

*Ingredients:*
100g of brown basmati rice, ¼ tablespoon of oil, ½ a small onion finely chopped, ½ a garlic clove chopped, ½ teaspoon of fennel seeds, ½ teaspoon of sesame seeds, ¼ teaspoon of ground turmeric, ½ teaspoon of ground cumin, pinch of salt, 1 whole clove, 2 cardamom pods lightly crushed, 2 black peppercorns, 225ml of chicken stock, fresh coriander to garnish

*Preparation:* Wash the rice well and leave to soak for 30 minutes. Heat a touch of oil in a heavy based saucepan and add the onion and garlic, gently fry for 5 minutes. Then, stir in the fennel seeds, turmeric, salt, cumin, cloves, cardamom pods and peppercorns and fry for a further minute. Drain the rice and then add to the pan and stir fry for 2 minutes.

Pour the chicken stock and bring to the boil. After this lower the heat and gently simmer for 15 minutes until the liquid has absorbed. Sprinkle with fresh coriander to serve.

* Brown Basmati Rice does need to be cooked for longer in comparison to white rice, so cooking time may vary

## Pea and Mushroom Pilau Rice                              High Carb
Nutritional Facts:  Carbs 45g, Saturated Fat 0.2g Unsaturated Fat 2.0g

*Ingredients:*
100g of brown basmati rice, ½ tablespoon of oil, ¼ teaspoon of cumin seeds, 1 black cardamom pod, 1 cinnamon stick, 1 garlic clove sliced, pinch of salt, ½ a

medium tomato, 25g of button mushrooms, 40g of petis pois, 400ml of water.

*Preparation:* First wash the rice and leave to soak for 30 minutes. In a heavy based saucepan heat the oil and add all the spices, garlic and pinch of salt. Add the tomato and mushrooms and stir fry for 2 minutes. Drain the rice and add to the pan with the peas stirring gently. Add water and bring to the boil. Lower the heat, cover and continue to cook for 10 minutes.

Pour the chicken stock and bring to the boil. After this lower the heat and gently simmer for 15 minutes until the liquid has absorbed. Sprinkle with fresh coriander to serve.

* Brown Basmati Rice does need to be cooked for longer in comparison to white rice, so cooking time may vary

## Tomato Rice     High Carb
Nutritional Facts: Carbs 45g, Saturated Fat 0.2g Unsaturated Fat 2.0g

*Ingredients:*
100g of brown basmati rice, ½ tablespoon of oil, ¼ teaspoon of onion seeds, ½ medium onion sliced, 1 medium tomato sliced, ½ yellow pepper, ¼ teaspoon of the following, ginger pulp, garlic pulp and chili powder, 1 tablespoon of fresh coriander, ½ medium potato sliced, pinch of salt, 25g of peas, 400ml of water

*Preparation:* First wash the rice and leave to soak for 30 minutes. In a heavy based saucepan heat the oil and fry the onion seeds for approximately 30 seconds. Add the sliced onion and fry for 3-4 minutes stirring to avoid them sticking to the pan. Add the tomatoes, pepper, ginger, chili powder, garlic, fresh coriander, potato, pinch of salt and peas and stir fry over medium heat for 4 minutes. After draining the rice add to the pan and stir fry for 2 minutes.

Pour in the water, bring to the boil and then lower the heat. Cover and leave for 10-12 minutes.

* Brown Basmati Rice does need to be cooked for longer in comparison to white rice, so cooking time may vary

## Vegetable Biryani                                    High Carb

Nutritional Facts:  Carbs 40g, Saturated Fat 0.1g Unsaturated Fat 1.0g

*Ingredients:*
100g of brown basmati rice, 1 whole clove, 1 cadamom pod (seeds only), 200ml of vegetable stock, 1 garlic clove, ½ a small onion chopped, ½ teaspoon of cumin seeds, ½ teaspoon of ground coriander, pinch of ground turmeric, pinch of chili powder, pinch of salt and black pepper, ½ a large potato, 1 sliced carrot, 2-3 small cauliflower florets, 25g of french or green beans or broccoli, 1 tablespoon of fresh coriander, 1 tablespoon of lime juice, fresh coriander to garnish

*Preparation:* Wash the rice and add the clove and cardamom seeds and pour into a heavy based saucepan. Pour in vegetable stock and bring to the boil. Then, reduce the heat, cover and allow to simmer for 15-20 minutes, until stock has absorbed.

Using a blender, add the garlic clove, onion, cumin seeds, ground coriander, turmeric, chili powder and remainder of spices into the blender or grinder and add 1-2 tablespoons of water and blend to a smooth paste.

Preheat oven to 180. Using the top shelf of the cooker add the spicy paste to a casserole dish and cook over low heat for 2 minutes, stirring to ensure it does not stick. Then, add the potato, cut into cubes, carrots, cauliflower and beans along with 4 tablespoons of water. Cover and cook for 12 minutes. Add the fresh coriander, remove the cloves from the rice and sprinkle with lime juice. Cover and cook for an additional 20 minutes until the vegetables are tender.

* Brown Basmati Rice does need to be cooked for longer in comparison to white rice

## Pea and Mushroom Pilau                              High Carb

Nutritional Facts: Protein 10g, Carbs 40g, Saturated Fat 0.4g, Unsaturated Fat 3.8g

*Ingredients:*
100g of basmati rice, touch of oil, pinch of cumin seeds, ½ a black cardamom pod, ½ a cinnamon stick, 1 garlic clove crushed, pinch of salt, ½ a medium tomato, handful of button mushrooms, handful of petis pois or tinned peas, 160ml of water

Leave the rice to soak for 30 minutes. Next, heat a little oil in a heavy based saucepan and begin frying all the spices and garlic. Then, add the tomato and mushrooms and continue frying for 2 minutes. Add a pinch of salt. Drain the rice and add to saucepan along with the peas. Add the water bringing to the boil. Then, cover, lower the heat and cook for a further 15 minutes.

## Rice with Lentils — High Carb

Nutritional Facts: Protein 7g, Carbs 35g, Saturated Fat 0.4g, Unsaturated Fat 3.8g

*Ingredients:*
60g of basmati rice, 40g of red split peas, ½ a medium potato, ½ a small onion, touch of oil, 1 clove, pinch of cumin seeds and ground turmeric, pinch of salt, 80ml of water

You can use tinned peas or fresh. If using fresh be sure to wash in cold water. Leave in bowl and cover with water and leave to soak for 10 minutes. Peel the potato and cut into chunks. Next, thinly slice the small onion and set aside. Using a heavy based saucepan, heat a little oil and fry the clove and cumin seeds until they splutter. Next, add the onion and potato and fry for 4 minutes. Add the lentils, rice, turmeric and pinch of salt and fry for a further 3 minutes. Lastly, add the water and bring to the boil, cover and simmer gently for 15 minutes until the water has absorbed.

## Jade Fried Rice — High Carb

Nutritional Facts:  Carbs 35g, Saturated Fat 0.2g Unsaturated Fat 1.4g

*Ingredients:*
100g of Brown Basmati Rice, 1 Garlic Clove, ¼ teaspoon of crushed ginger, 1 medium sized zuccini/courgette sliced, 1 medium carrot sliced, 10 spinach leaves, ½ tablespoon of oil, 1 tablespoon soy sauce, pinch of salt, pinch of pepper

*Preparation:* First wash the zuccini and cut into cubes, same with the carrot and spinach which should be chopped into pieces. Wash and soak the rice for 30 minutes, then using a heavy based saucepan, add a little oil and stiry fry the garlic and ginger for 1 minute. Then, add the carrot, zuccini and stir fry for an additional 2 minutes. Add the spinach, soy sauce and rice and cook for an additional minute. Season with touch of salt and pepper.

* Brown Basmati Rice does need to be cooked for longer in comparison to white rice, so cooking time may vary

# BUILDING YOUR **BEST** BODY

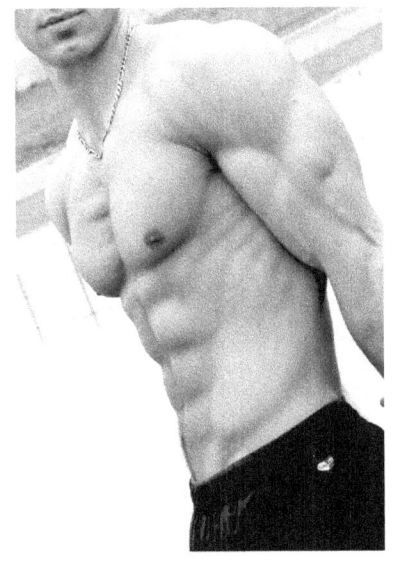

It's a fact that resistance placed on all muscle groups such as the biceps, triceps, chest, legs and shoulders will actually benefit your abdominals. A good balanced weight-training program will actually **burn fat cells**, **speed up the metabolic rate** and of course **create a well-proportioned physique.** You can have a great set of abs, but wouldn't it be nice to compliment them with bigger biceps, a chiseled chest and toned legs, to complete the picture? The Lean Muscle Plan is going to provide you with an all round body conditioner to give you that *Total Body Makeover!*

## PROGRAM INTRODUCTION

The achievement of a superb, lean physique is obviously the main goal of anyone interested in fitness and body-building. Any successful training program certainly requires commitment and determination and must always start with an understanding of the basics - muscular size and strength. Simply put, to increase lean muscle, it must be increased in strength. The well known saying: "The strength of a muscle is in direct proportion to its size." could not be more true.

There comes a point where muscles can be exercised without changing their form. Going beyond this point will have a direct and marked effect on lean muscular growth. However, it should be remembered that it's the quality and intensity of an exercise that matters - not how much is done. If any particular exercise falls below a certain level of intensity, the muscle will simply not increase in size. The higher intensity, the faster the muscular size and strength increase.

## EXERCISE INTENSITY

The understanding of 'intensity' often poses problems for trainees. Intensity is not related either to the amount of work you are doing or to the production of power. In basic terms it is a reflection of the percentage of momentary ability actually being used. Maximum intensity means you are using as much muscular force to perform an exercise as possible at any given moment.

During exercise, levels of intensity constantly fluctuate. It's not always possible to perform an exercise to maximum intensity due to the fatigue your muscles have experienced on a previous exercise. Experts believe that intensity levels of 100% are the fastest way to build muscle size and strength. But how do you know if you are producing this level of intensity?

The only way to ensure you are reaching full intensity is to reach the point of **MMF (Momentary Muscular Failure).**

**Momentary Muscular Failure:** The point of an exercise at which you have so fully fatigued the working muscles that they can no longer complete an additional repetition of a movement with strict form.

Basically if you have performed as many repetitions for any given exercise and find that lifting one more repetition is impossible, then you have reached 100% level of intensity. This also means that the muscles involved in the exercise have been worked to Momentary Muscular Failure and have been stimulated to optimum levels. Should you stop short by a few repetitions of intensity then you will not reach MMF and you will have stopped short of the threshold leading to lean muscular growth. In a nutshell, intensity is the key to success here, reach it and you'll force those muscles to grow, fall short of it and the muscles will have no stimulus to grow on.

This High-Intensity exercise is what will place the necessary demands on your muscles to increase in muscular size and strength. This exercise program will also increase strength and overall ability in other physical activities, and generally creates a feeling of well-being. Unfortunately the reverse effect can often happen and the trainee can be left feeling tired, drained and without energy. Obviously you will feel tired at the end of your first few workouts if you are new to exercise and weight lifting, but if the feeling persists it is a clear indication that you are over training. Workouts should never exceed the recovery ability of the body.

High-intensity exercise places enormous demands on the body that are not easily met. A muscle being worked very hard requires vast quantities of oxygen and nutrition and the quality training program will not have the full effect without proper diet and lifestyle. When exercise is completed it is vitally important the muscles are given sufficient time to return to normal. Muscular growth and recuperation occur during periods of rest, therefore, failure to rest your muscles and continuing with high-intensity work to soon after your previous workout will result in muscle deterioration and loss in both muscle strength and size. I recommend at least 24 hours rest before hitting the weight again.

## QUALITY - NOT QUANTITY

This is a very common misconception that an increase in the amount of exercise done will automatically lead to an increase in the intensity of the exercise. Not only is this completely wrong but it will drastically impede your progress. The minimum amount of exercise that causes the greatest amount of growth stimulation will always produce the very best results. If the program is going to work for you then the load must be heavy enough to force muscles to work. Before a muscle is capable of its maximum effort it must first be warmed up through the repetition several times by a movement lighter than it is capable of handling. Cold muscles fail at a level far below their actual strength. Isometric exercises (Stretching exercises) simply don't provide sufficient stimulation to force muscles to work inside their existing levels of strength reserve. This is not to say that isometrics have no place in a body-building program. Far from it! Isometric contractions (Stretches – See Page 164should terminate every set of almost every exercise - after the maximum number of full movements has been performed. At this stage - say in the eleventh or twelfth repetition, the muscles will fail completely and although they may be contracting as hard as possible against a heavy resistance no movement will occur. This indicates that an exercise has been properly terminated and maximum growth stimulation reached.

## FORM

To witness the maximum benefits of the Lean Muscle Plan, performance style is of crucial importance. Proper form includes the following:

## ISOLATION MOVEMENT

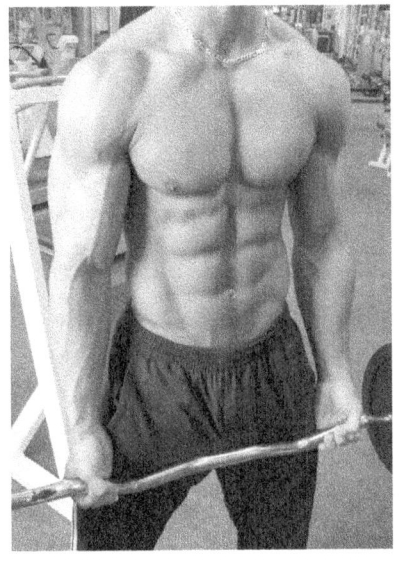

This is an exercise involving only one muscle group or part of the body; it involves a single joint rotary movement. The trainee should, regardless of the particular exercise or equipment being used, concentrate on isolating only the muscles used in a specific movement, doing as many repetitions as possible in perfect form. Cheating - bringing surrounding muscles into action should be avoided. Only in compound exercises, when no other perfect repetitions can be performed, is cheating permissible - but even then it should be kept at an absolute minimum.

## RELAXATION OF UNINVOLVED MUSCLES

The isolation of a particular muscle is directly related to the ability to relax the uninvolved muscles. Dangerous levels of stress may be reached if the trainee places too much stress on too many muscles simultaneously. A warning sign of this is the development of headaches during exercise. Greater energy, and therefore more efficient growth stimulation, can be released to the isolated muscle if you learn to effectively relax your other body parts.

## RANGE OF MOVEMENT

A fully contracting muscle produces a full range of movement. If a particular movement is less than full range, the entire length of the muscle will not be involved in the work. In order to achieve the desired effect of increased lean muscular shape and size, the range of movement of each repetition should be as great as possible.

## SUPERVISION

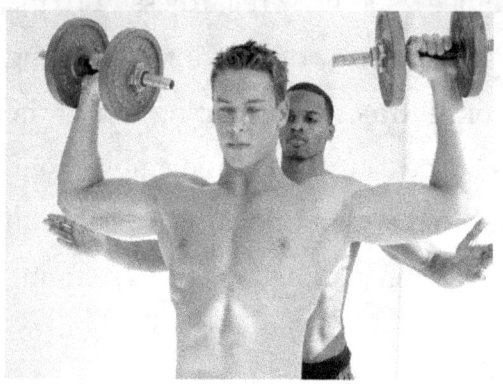

High-intensity exercise, properly performed, is very demanding and few people find it possible to workout effectively with out the use of a training partner or spotter. The presence of a supervisor acts as encouragement and inspiration. *A spotter is recommended with Squats and Bench Presses.*

## WORKOUTS - How many, How Often?

This a question which could be disputed forever. Unfortunately this confusion is still fairly widespread and results in many people spending as many as 20 hours a week training, in an attempt to accelerate progress, when in fact better results would be produced if they limited their training to not more than three hours of correct exercise per week. The actual time needed to develop lean muscle size is not that great, and this is a vital fact that all trainees must understand. It should also be pointed out that once any high intensity workout has been completed, the body needs approximately 24-48 hours to renew itself. Therefore beginners should not train on consecutive days. This plan recommends a three day training routine every other day. Monday, Wednesday and Friday and an optional workout on Saturday or Sunday.

## PERFORMING EXERCISES

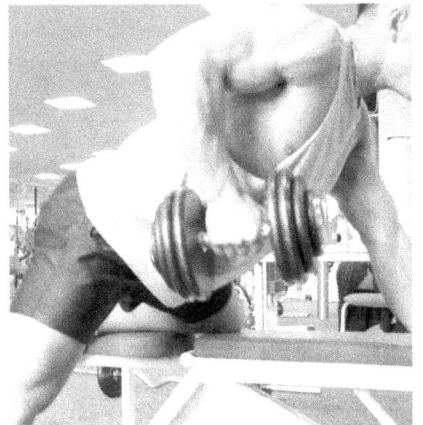 The range of movement and control of each exercise is very important. Jerking the weight or using other muscle groups should be avoided. A simple guideline is the following: it should take two seconds to lift the weight and four to lower it, or in other words, two seconds positive and four seconds negative. Not only does doing exercises in this way decrease the amount of weight used, but it vastly increases results, as well as almost totally eliminating the chance of injury. Exercise concentrated on one particular muscle will also have an effect, albeit to a lesser degree on other muscles of the body, even those not being exercised at all. An unbalanced exercise program will, to a certain extent, develop certain muscles disproportionately, but the body seems to impose its own limits on this unbalanced development.

## EXERCISE SEQUENCE

A number of important conclusions can be drawn from the effect concept.

- Best results will be achieved only if the training program is properly balanced and includes exercises for each of the major muscle groups.

- Greater emphasis should be placed on working the largest muscle groups of the body. The Lean Muscle plan will involve a split routine, training two body parts on each workout, i.e., chest and biceps on a Monday. Each body part will be trained once weekly.

## Chest & Biceps    MONDAY

1. **Upper Abs Routine**

2. **Bench Press** x 3 sets

3. **Pec Deck or Dumbbell Flyes** x 3 sets

4. **Cable Crossovers or Incline Dumbbell Press** x 2 sets

5. **Dumbbell Curls** x 3 sets

6. **Barbell Curls** x 3 sets

7. **Concentration Curls** x 2 sets

8. **10 minutes Cardio** (LOW INTENSITY)
   **Week 2 - 12 minutes**

## Shoulders & Triceps    WEDS

1. **Oblique Abs Routine**

2. **Shoulder Press** x 3 sets

3. **Front Raises** x 3 sets

4. **Shoulder Raises** x 2 sets

5. **Close Grip Bench Press** x 3 sets

6. **Kickbacks** x 3 sets

7. **Tricep Extension** x 2 sets

8. **10 minutes Cardio** (LOW INTENSITY)
   **Week 2 - 12 minutes**

## Legs & Back    FRIDAY

1. **Lower Abs Routine**

2. **Leg Extension** x 3 sets

3. **Smith Machine Squats** x 2 sets

4. **Hamstring Curls** x 3 sets

\* **Optional: Calf Raises** x 3 sets

5. **Lat Pulldown** x 3 sets

6. **Barbell Rows** x 3 sets

7. **Dumbbell Rows** x 3 sets

### NOTES WK 1:

- Workout Day may change according to your schedule.

- Aim for a weight in which you can comfortably lift more than 6 reps, but begin to fail around 12. If you find you can perform more than 15 reps comfortably, increase the poundage.

- Increase the poundage on each set, for example: Set 1: 10kg, Set 2, 15kg, Set 3 17.5 kg.

- Low Intensity Cardio may be substituted for High Intensity Cardio, however, please half the time.

**HIGH CARB DAY**

### NOTES Continued:

- As I recommend between 4-6 sessions of cardio weekly (4 for complete beginners) you will need to add an additional two sessions as no cardio should be performed after legs. Two morning sessions would be recommended.

- Stretching after each exercise is very important. Please ensure you stretch after each set (see page 118) for approximately 8-10 seconds.

- Ensure you stick to the principle of two seconds to lift the weight and four seconds to lower it.

**HIGH-MOD CARB DAY**

### NOTES Continued:

- If you are limited to the equipment you have access to be sure to use some of the other exercises outlined in the book.

- Don't over do it on your first week, just use this week to get used to the exercises.

- Keep rest periods short. No more than 30 seconds between each set and 1 minute between different exercises.

**HIGH CARB DAY**

## Chest & Biceps  **MONDAY**

1. **Upper Abs Routine** (See Page 182) **WK5**: (Page 183)
2. **Incline Bench Press** x 3 sets
3. **Dumbbell Flyes** x 3 sets
4. **Flat Dumbbell Press** x 3 sets
5. **Cable Crossovers** x 2 sets
6. **Barbell Curls** x 3 sets
7. **Preacher Curls** x 3 sets
8. **Hammer Curls** x 3 sets
9. **Concentration Curls** x 2 sets

10. **14 minutes Cardio**
(LOW INTENSITY)

**Week 4 - 15 minutes, Week 5 & 6 - 16 minutes**

### NOTES WK 3 - 6:

- Workout Day may change according to your schedule.

- Increase the poundage on each set, for example: Set 1: 10kg, Set 2, 15kg, Set 3 17.5 kg.

- Aim for failure on your last two sets of each exercise. Failure should set it at around 6-8 reps, so you will need to find a weight heavy enough. If you find you can comfortably lift more than 12 reps, you should increase the weight.

*HIGH CARB DAY*

## Shoulders & Triceps  **WEDS**

1. **Oblique Abs Routine** (See Page 182) **WK5**: (Page 183)
2. **Dumbbell Press** x 3 sets
3. **Upright Row** x 3 sets
4. **Smith Machine Press** x 3 sets
5. **Shoulder Raises** x 2 sets
6. **Cable Extensions** x 3 sets
7. **Close Grip Press** x 3 sets
8. **Tricep Extension** x 3 sets
9. **Skull Crushers** x 2 sets

10. **14 minutes Cardio**
(LOW INTENSITY)

**Week 4 - 15 minutes, Week 5 & 6 - 16 minutes**

### NOTES Continued:

- As I recommend between 4-6 sessions of cardio weekly you will need to add an additional two sessions as no cardio should be performed after legs. Two morning sessions would be recommended.

- Continue stretching after each exercise. Please ensure you stretch after each set (see page 118) for approximately 8-10 seconds.

- Ensure you stick to the principle of two seconds to lift the weight and four seconds to lower it.

*HIGH-MOD CARB DAY*

## Legs & Back  **FRIDAY**

1. **Lower Abs Routine** (See Page 182) **WK5**: (Page 183)
2. **Leg Extension** x 3 sets
3. **Smith Machine Squats** x 2 sets
4. **Lunges** x 3 sets
5. **Hamstring Curls** x 3 sets
6. **Wide Grip Pull Ups** x 3 sets
7. **Reverse Grip Barbell Rows** x 3 sets
8. **Cable Rows** x 3 sets
9. **Lat Pulldown** x 2 sets

### NOTES Continued:

- If you are limited to the equipment you have access to be sure to use some of the other exercises outlined in the book.

- If you're limited with time, you can train your abs earlier or on different days.

- Keep rest periods short. No more than 25 seconds between each set and 50 seconds between different exercises.

*HIGH CARB DAY*

# The **Bollywood Workout** Plan Week 7 - 10

## Chest & Biceps — MONDAY

1. **Upper Abs Routine**
2. **Flat Bench Press** x 4 sets
3. **Incline Dumbbell Flyes** x 3 sets
4. **Decline Bench Press** x 3 sets
5. **Peck Deck** x 3 sets
6. **Dumbbell Curls** x 3 sets
7. **EZ Bar Curls** x 3 sets
8. **Cable Curls** x 3 sets
9. **Concentration Curls** x 2 sets
10. **17 minutes Cardio** (LOW INTENSITY)

**Week 8 - 17 minutes, Week 9 & 10 - 18 minutes**

## Shoulders & Triceps — WEDS

1. **Oblique Abs Routine**
2. **Smith Machine Press** x 3 sets
3. **Side Raises** x 3 sets
4. **Front Raises** x 3 sets
5. **Upright Row** x 3 sets
6. **Cable Extensions** x 3 sets
7. **EZ Bar Close Press** x 3 sets
8. **Overhead Extension** x 3 sets
9. **Kickbacks** x 3 sets
10. **17 minutes Cardio** (LOW INTENSITY)

**Week 8 - 17 minutes, Week 9 & 10 - 18 minutes**

## Legs & Back — FRIDAY

1. **Lower Abs Routine**
2. **Leg Extension** x 3 sets
3. **Leg Press Machine** x 3 sets
4. **Lunges** x 3 sets
5. **Hamstring Curls** x 3 sets
6. **Wide Grip Pull Ups** x 3 sets
7. **Wide Grip Pull Down** x 3 sets
8. **V-Bar Cable Rows** x 3 sets
9. **One Arm Rows** x 2 sets

## NOTES WK 7-10:

- Workout Day may change according to your schedule.

- You will now implement a pyramid system with your exercises whereby you increase the poundage on each set and then lower back to a light weight on Set 4, for example:
  Set 1: 30kg, Set 2: 40kg, Set 3: 50kg, Set 4: 30kg

- Continue to work to failure on your last three sets. The 1st Set is your warm up in which you should aim for 12 reps.

### HIGH CARB DAY

## NOTES Continued:

- As I recommend between 4-6 sessions of cardio weekly you will need to add an additional two sessions as no cardio should be performed after legs. Two morning sessions would be recommended.

- Continue stretching after each exercise. Please ensure you stretch after each set (see page 118) for approximately 8-10 seconds.

- Ensure you stick to the principle of two seconds to lift the weight and four seconds to lower it.

### HIGH-MOD CARB DAY

## NOTES Continued:

- If you are limited to the equipment you have access to be sure to use some of the other exercises outlined in the book.

- If you're limited with time, you can train your abs earlier or on different days.

- Keep rest periods short. No more than 25 seconds between each set and 50 seconds between different exercises.

### HIGH CARB DAY

## Chest & Biceps — MONDAY

1. **Upper Abs Routine**
2. **Decline Bench Press** x 4 sets
3. **Dumbbell Flyes** x 3 sets
4. **Incline Dumbbell Press** x 3 sets
5. **Cable Crossovers** x 3 sets
6. **EZ Bar Curls** x 3 sets
7. **Close Grip Cable Curls** x 3 sets
8. **Concentration Curls** x 3 sets
9. **Hammer Curls** x 3 sets
10. **18 minutes Cardio** (LOW INTENSITY)

**Week 12 - 20 minutes**

### NOTES WK 11-12:

- Workout Day may change according to your schedule.

- You will now implement a pyramid system with your exercises whereby you increase the poundage on each set and then lower back to a light weight on Set 4, for example:
Set 1: 30kg, Set 2: 40kg, Set 3: 50kg, Set 4: 30kg

- Continue to work to failure on your last three sets. The 1st Set is your warm up in which you should aim for 12 reps.

*HIGH CARB DAY*

## Shoulders & Triceps — WEDS

1. **Oblique Abs Routine**
2. **Dumbbell Press** x 3 sets
3. **Upright Row** x 3 sets
4. **Front Raises** x 3 sets
5. **Side Cable Raises** x 3 sets
6. **Close Grip Press** x 3 sets
7. **EZ Bar Close Press** x 3 sets
8. **Cable Extensions** x 3 sets
9. **Kickbacks** x 3 sets
10. **18 minutes Cardio** (LOW INTENSITY)

**Week 12 - 20 minutes**

### NOTES Continued:

- As I recommend between 4-6 sessions of cardio weekly you will need to add an additional two sessions as no cardio should be performed after legs. Two morning sessions would be recommended.

- Continue stretching after each exercise. Please ensure you stretch after each set (see page 118) for approximately 8-10 seconds.

- Ensure you stick to the principle of two seconds to lift the weight and four seconds to lower it.

*HIGH-MOD CARB DAY*

## Legs & Back — FRIDAY

1. **Lower Abs Routine**
2. **Smith Machine Squats** x 3 sets
3. **Leg Press Machine** x 3 sets
4. **Leg Extensions** x 3 sets
5. **Hamstring Curls** x 3 sets
6. **Close Grip Pull Down** x 3 sets
7. **Reverse Grip Barbell Rows** x 3 sets
8. **Wide Grip Cable Rows** x 3 sets
9. **One Arm Rows or Gym Lat Machine** x 3 sets

### NOTES Continued:

- If you are limited to the equipment you have access to be sure to use some of the other exercises outlined in the book.

- If you're limited with time, you can train your abs earlier or on different days.

- Keep rest periods short. No more than 25 seconds between each set and 50 seconds between different exercises.

*HIGH CARB DAY*

# The **Bollywood Workout** Advanced Program

## Chest & Biceps

### MONDAY

1. **Upper Abs Routine**
2. **Bench Press** x 4 sets
3. **Decline Dumbbell Flyes** x 4 sets
4. **Incline Bench Press** x 4 sets
5. **Cable Crossovers** x 3 sets
6. **EZ Bar Curls** x 4 sets
7. **Close Grip Cable Curls** x 4 sets
8. **Dumbbell Curls** x 4 sets
9. **Concentration Curls** x 3 sets
10. **20 minutes Cardio**
   (LOW INTENSITY)

### NOTES ADVANCED PROGRAM:

- Workout Days may change according to your schedule.

- Use the pyramid system with your exercises whereby you increase the poundage on each set and then lower back to a light weight on Set 4, for example:
  Set 1: 30kg, Set 2: 40kg, Set 3: 50kg, Set 4: 30kg

- Work to failure on your last three sets. The 1st Set is your warm up in which you should aim for 12 reps.

*HIGH CARB DAY*

## Shoulders & Triceps

### WEDS

1. **Oblique Abs Routine**
2. **Dumbbell Press** x 4 sets
3. **Upright Row** x 4 sets
4. **Barbell Front Raises** x 4 sets
5. **Side Raises** x 3 sets
6. **Close Grip Press** x 4 sets
7. **EZ Bar Close Press** x 4 sets
8. **Cable Extensions** x 4 sets
9. **Kickbacks** x 3 sets
10. **18 minutes Cardio**
   (LOW INTENSITY)

### NOTES Continued:

- I recommend between 4-6 sessions of cardio weekly so you will need to add an additional two or more sessions as no cardio should be performed after legs. Morning sessions would be recommended.

- Please ensure you stretch after each set (see page 118) for approximately 8-10 seconds.

- Ensure you stick to the principle of two seconds to lift the weight and four seconds to lower it.

*HIGH-MOD CARB DAY*

## Legs & Back

### FRIDAY

1. **Lower Abs Routine**
2. **Smith Machine Squats** x 4 sets
3. **Leg Press Machine** x 4 sets
4. **Leg Extensions** x 4 sets
5. **Hamstring Curls** x 3 sets
6. **Close Grip Pull Down** x 4 sets
7. **Reverse Grip Barbell Rows** x 4 sets
8. **Wide Grip Cable Rows** x 4 sets
9. **One Arm Rows or Gym Lat Machine** x 3 sets

### NOTES Continued:

- If you are limited to the equipment you have access to be sure to use some of the other exercises outlined in the book.

- If you're limited with time, you can train your abs earlier or on different days.

- Keep rest periods short. No more than 25 seconds between each set and 50 seconds between different exercises.

*HIGH CARB DAY*

# High Intensity
## Fat Burner Workout

The following workout is a great fat burning workout which is very intensive and should only be undertaken by Intermediate or Advanced Trainees. You can use this routine as a plateau breaker every five weeks for a whole week just to mix things up and encourage new growth and increase fat loss. Alternatively you may use this program as your main workout routine.

**Here are the workouts split up:**

**Monday:** Chest and Biceps with Upper Abs and HIIT

**Tuesday:** Shoulders and Triceps with HIIT

**Thursday:** Cardio, Legs and Obliques

**Friday:** HIIT, Back and Lower Abs

**Saturday or Sunday** - Additional 1-2 Cardio Sessions

Ok, now let's look at this workout in more detail.

**Mondays Session:**

Begin with a 3 minute warm up (50% of your maximum) on any piece of cardio apparatus and then immediately move onto Abs. Today you will work upper abs so choose one exercise of your choice and perform three sets.

Without resting I'd like you to move straight onto your Chest Exercises (three exercises for three sets). Immediately following your chest exercises please then move onto your upper abs again, choosing two different exercises and again perform three sets for each.

Having finished your abs, I'd like you to move back onto a cardio machine of your choice for a further 3 minutes of cardio at approximately 50% effort. Once finished, please then move onto your bicep exercises, again choose three exercises and perform three sets.

Once you've finished your workout, you will end it with cardio (10 minutes in duration). You can either perform HIIT or Low Intensity (60-75% maximum effort).

The above workout is a real fat burner as it combines both cardio and resistance exercise and it must be performed with very little rest (this ensures you keep your heart rate elevated).

Exercises to choose from:

**CHEST**
- Cable Crossover machine (light weight)
- Incline Barbell Press
- Incline Cable Flyes
- Flat Bench Dumbbell Press
- Decline Press
- Cable Crossovers or Pec Deck

**BICEPS**
- Barbell Curls
- Dumbbell Curls
- Concentration Curls

- Cable Curls
- Close Grip EZ Bar Curls

**Tuesdays Session.**

Again, begin your workout with the 3 minute warm up on a piece of cardio apparatus. Once you've finished, move onto your shoulder workout, choosing three exercises and performing three sets.

Once finished move back onto a piece of cardio equipment, ideally something different than which you began your workout with. This time you will perform 8 minutes of HIIT (Page 212

Having completed the 8 minute HIIT workout you will move onto your tricep workout where you should pick three exercises for three sets.

On completion of the above you should then return to the cardio apparatus to complete your workout with a further 10 minute HIIT session. This will complete Tuesdays workout.

**SHOULDERS**
- Upright Row
- Smith Machine Press
- Front Raises
- Lateral Side Raises

**TRICEPS**
- Dips
- Tricep Extension
- Rope Pushdown
- Kickbacks

- Straight Bar Pushdown

**Wednesday should be an 'off' day.**

**Thursdays Workout**

I'd like you to begin this session with a 10 minute cardio session (50% maximum effort) to warm up those legs before the workout. I'd especially recommend either the stationery bike or elliptical machine.

On completion of your cardio please move onto your oblique ab exercise. Please pick one exercise and perform three sets. Once done it is time to move onto your leg training, pick three exercises and perform three sets. On the last set of each of your exercises, you should reduce the weight and perform an increased amount of repetitions (between 10-20).

Having completed the leg workout, please then move onto the final part of your oblique training, this time choose two exercises and perform three sets for each. This completes your Thursday session.

Exercises to choose from:

**LEGS**
- Squats on Smith Machine (shoulder width stance)
- Leg Press with feet close together
- Squat Rack (Duck squat position, toes pointing outwards)
- Leg Extensions
- Hamstring Curls
- Straight Leg Deadlifts with barbell or dumbbells
- Seated Calf Machine
- Leg Press

## Friday Workout

Fridays session begins with 8 minutes of HIIT on a piece of cardio equipment of your choice. After doing this you should then move onto your first lower ab exercise, choosing one exercise and performing three sets.

It is then time to move onto your back training, choosing three exercises and performing three sets for each. On the last set, please reduce the weight and increase the repetitions (10-20).

After this, please then move back to the ab training, with two lower exercises of your choice for three sets each.

To complete the workout you will perform 14 minutes of HIIT.

Exercises to choose from:

**BACK**

- Close Grip Lat Pulldown
- Wide Grip Behind Neck Pulldown
- Bent Over Row
- Machine Pull Back
- One Arm Row
- Deadlifts
- Hyperextensions

You can also add any additional cardio over the weekend if you would like to. Men can increase the sets to four per exercise or increase the number of exercises to four.

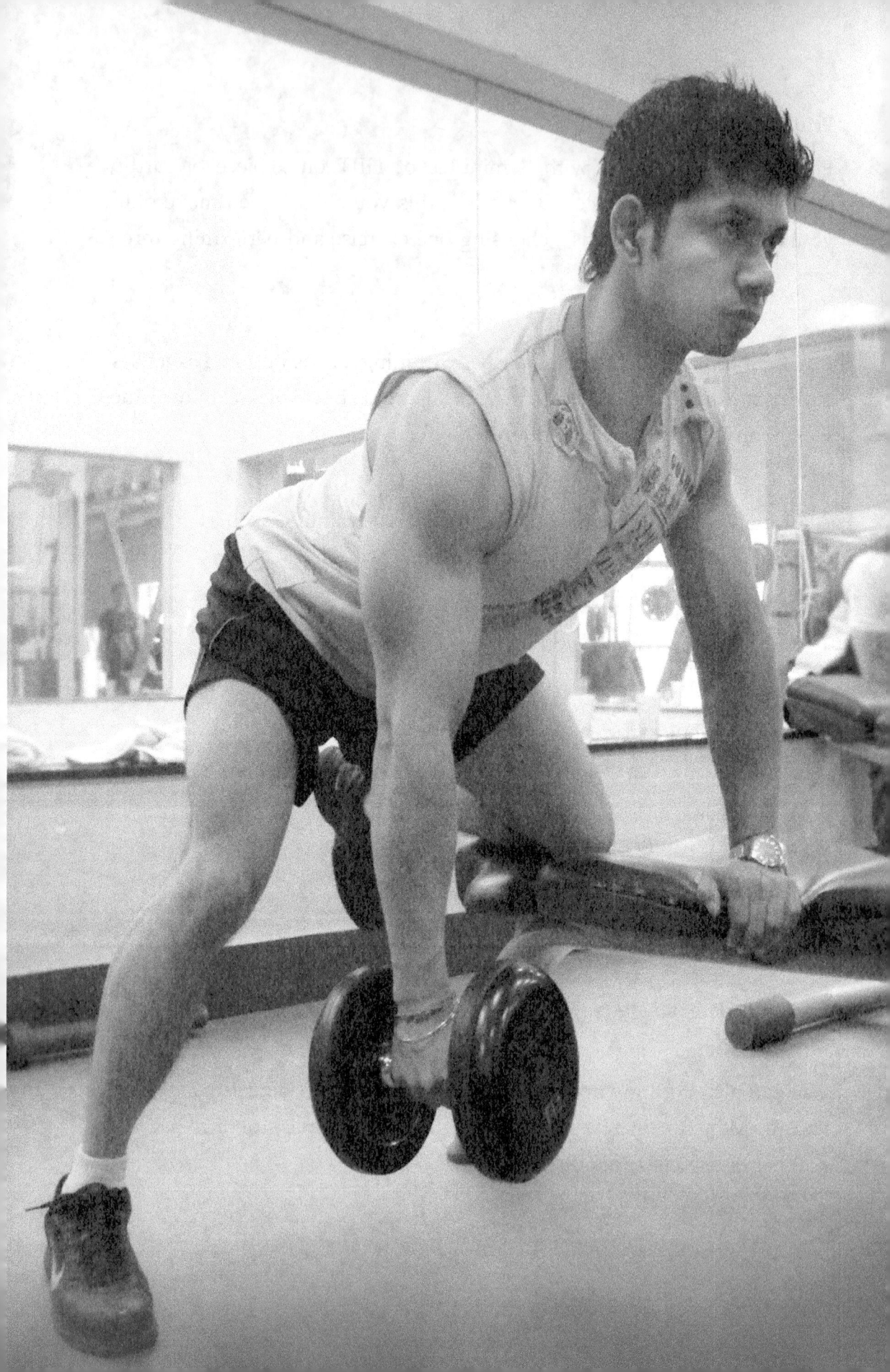

# **EXERCISE** GLOSSARY

## **Chest** Exercises

**Bench Press**

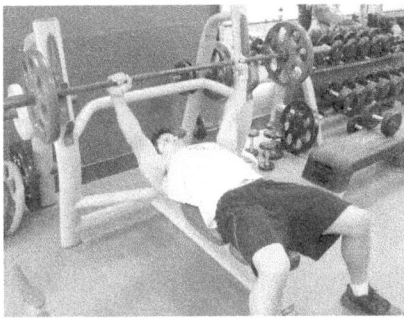 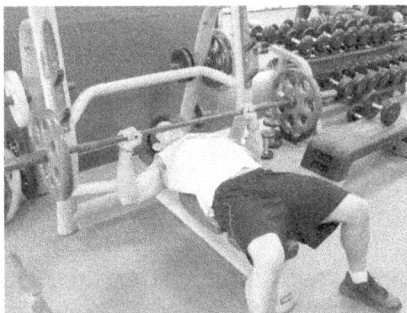

Position yourself on a flat bench. Lie flat on your back and grab the barbell above you with a grip slightly beyond shoulder width apart. Lift the barbell off of the rack and slowly lower it to about 3 inches above your chest and then press the bar back to the start position. Avoid touching the bar on your chest (this causes unneeded stress on your shoulder joints and takes the tension away from your chest muscles). Be sure that when you are lowering the bar that you do so in a slow and controlled fashion. Conversely, when you press the bar upward, you should do so in an explosive fashion. Repeat this movement for as many repetitions as you can until failure. Using a spotter on this exercise is very important just in case you fail and you're unable to re-rack the barbell.

## Peck Deck Fly

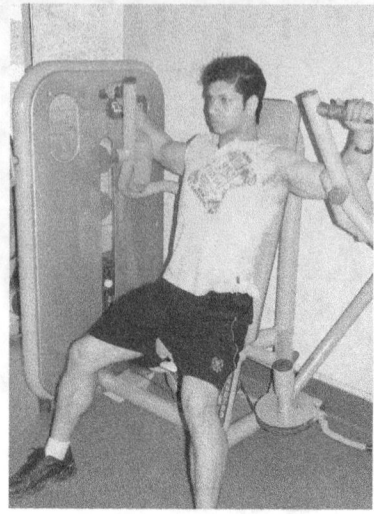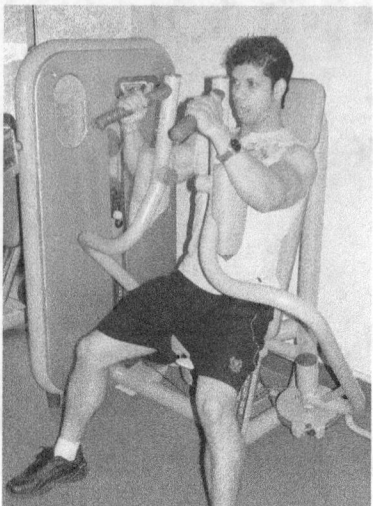

Using a Pec Deck machine, seat yourself in it and raise or lower the seat so that the fly grips are in line with your chest. Perform the exercise by squeezing your forearms and elbows in together so that you virtually touch them together at the peak of the movement. Be sure to really squeeze your chest at the peak of this movement for a one-count. Return to the start position and repeat.

## Dumbbell Press

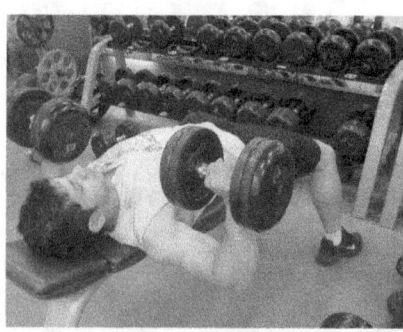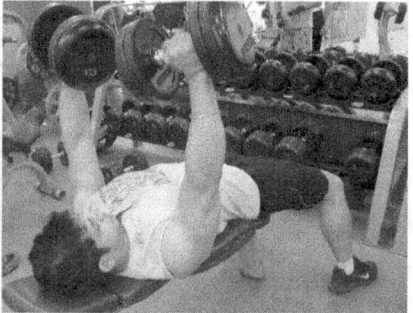

Lie flat on your back on a flat bench. With a dumbbell in each hand slowly press them upward and together. When you press them upward, you want to do so in an explosive fashion, just like the bench press. But when you lower the dumbbells you do so slowly and controlled.

## Dumbbell Fly

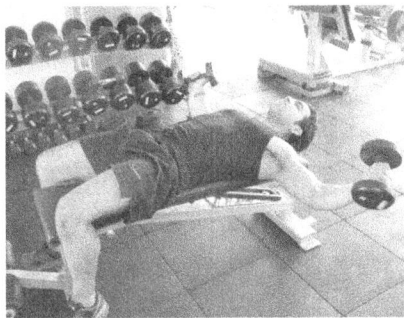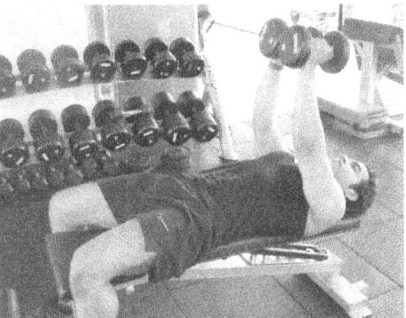

Position yourself on flat bench, flat on your back. With a dumbbell in each hand you should begin this movement with your arms stretched out wide to your sides with your elbows slightly bent and your palms facing inward, toward one another. When you lift the dumbbells up together, visualize hugging a giant tree trunk. At the peak of the movement, really squeeze your pecs together for a count of one. When returning to the start position, be sure to lower the dumbbells in a slow and controlled fashion. This exercise can also be performed on a decline (lower pecs) and incline (upper pecs).

## Decline Press

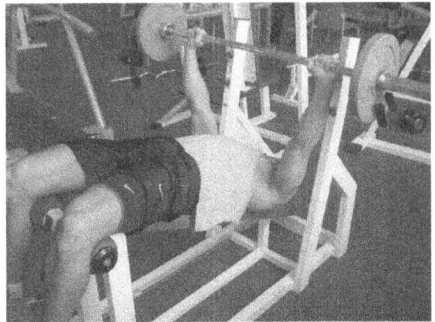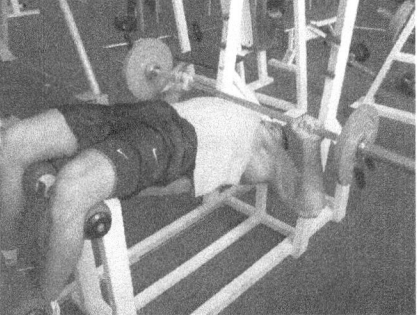

Position yourself on a decline bench and grab the barbell above you with a grip that is slightly beyond shoulder width apart. Lift the barbell off of the rack and slowly lower it to your chest and then press the bar back to the start position. Because of the angle of this exercise, touching the bar to your chest is actually ok with this exercise as doing so does not cause unneeded stress on your shoulders nor does it take the emphasis away from having your pecs do the work. Be sure that when you are lowering the bar that you do so in a slow and controlled fashion. Conversely, when you press the bar upward, you want to do so in an explosive fashion.

**Cable Crossovers**

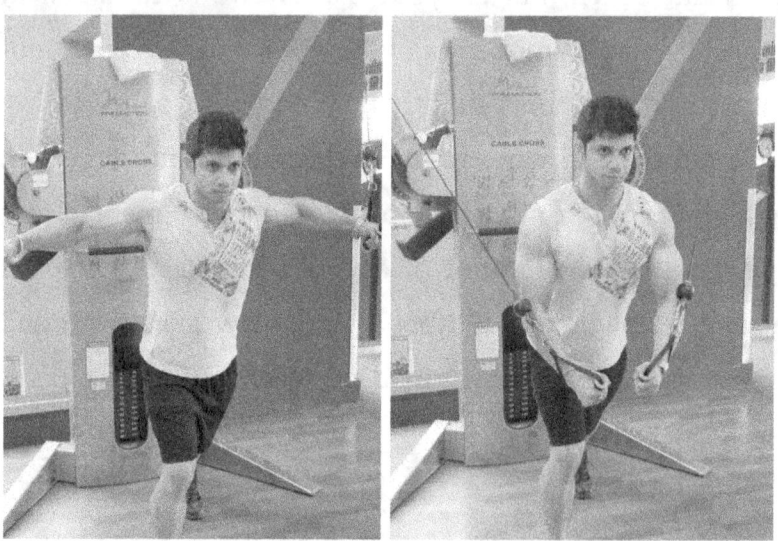

This exercise is performed using the cable pulley machine that has a pulley on two opposite sides. Set each pulley up so that it is locked in the high position. Stand in the middle and perpendicular to both pulleys. While standing, grab each high pulley using a small one-hand attachment for each hand. Slowly bring your arms together in a slow and controlled fashion. While doing so, visualize that you are hugging a giant tree trunk. At the peak of this movement, really flex your pec muscles together for a one-count and then return to the start position and repeat.

## Incline Dumbbell Press

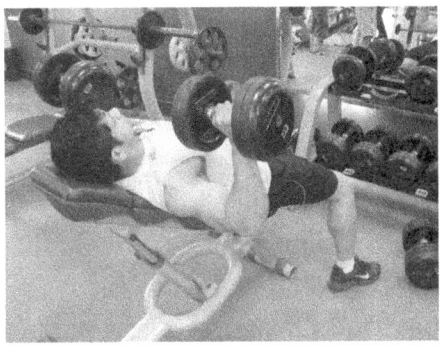

Performed exactly the same as the Flat Bench Dumbbell Press as shown on page 126. Grab each dumbbell using a regular grip instead of a grip where your palms face inward. Position yourself lying flat on an incline bench. With a dumbbell in each hand press the dumbbells upward in an explosive fashion. Then, return to the start position in a slow and controlled fashion. Repeat the movement for as many repetitions as you can until failure.

## Incline Bench Press

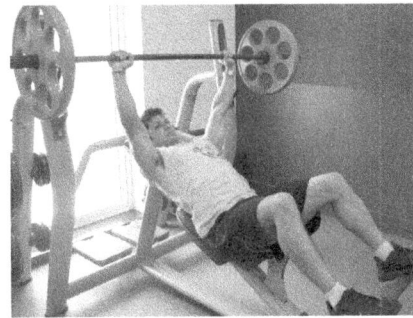 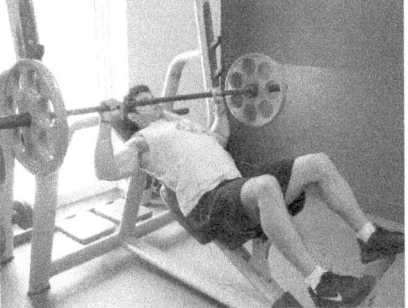

This exercise is very similar to the regular flat bench press except that you will be using an incline bench and your upper chest will be the muscle group worked instead of your middle chest. Lift the barbell off of the rack and slowly lower it to about three inches just below your Adam's Apple. Then, press the bar back to the start position. When you press the bar upward, you want to do so in an explosive fashion just like all the other press movements that have been covered. Repeat this movement for as many repetitions as you can until failure.

**Smith Machine Press**

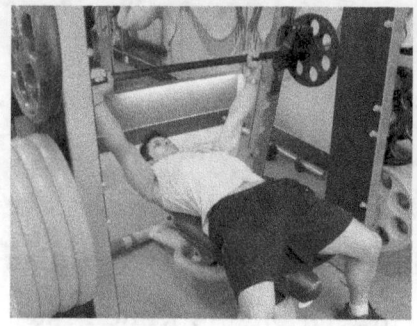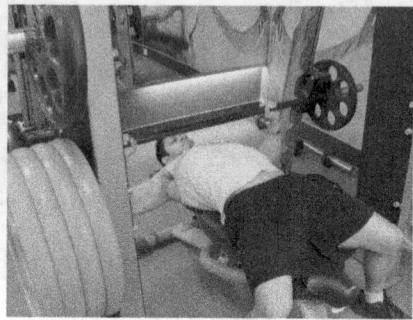

This exercise is very similar to the regular flat bench press. The only difference is that the Smith Machine acts as a spotter for you and is a safer alternative for trainees working out at home or on their own. Place a flat bench under a Smith Machine. Lie flat on your back and grab the barbell above you with a grip slightly beyond shoulder width apart. Lift the barbell off of the rack and slowly lower it to about three inches above your chest and then press the bar back to the start position.

# **Bicep** Exercises

### Dumbbell Curls

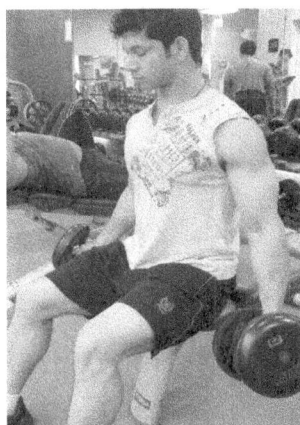 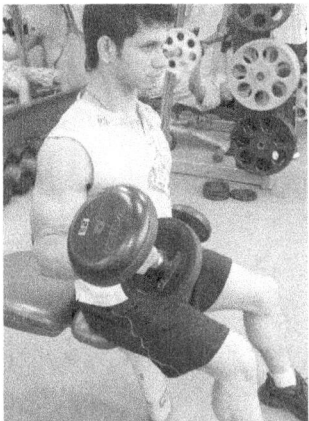

Sit at the end of a bench with your feet flat on the floor and your back upright and straight. Grabbing a dumbbell in each hand, let them hang at your sides with both palms facing inward toward the bench. Simultaneously curl the dumbbells up while twisting (i.e., supinating) your wrists outward on the way up. Be sure to squeeze your biceps at the top for a one-count.

### Barbell Curls

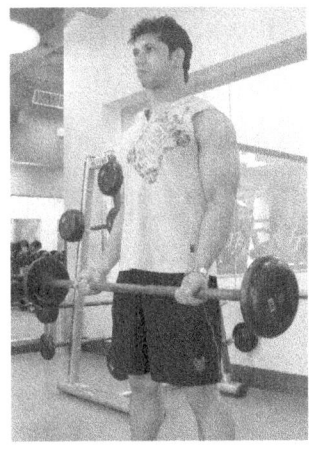 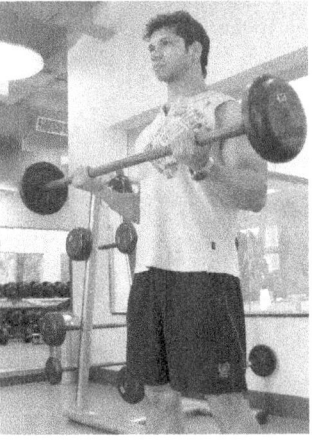

With your hands shoulder-width apart, grip a barbell with an underhand grip. Stand straight up with your shoulders squared and with your feet shoulder-width apart. Let the bar hang down at arm's length in front of you, with your arms, shoulders and hands in a straight line. Without leaning back or swinging the weight, curl the bar up toward your chest in an arc. Keep your elbows in the same place and close to your sides. Bring the weight up as high as you can and squeeze the biceps at the top. Lower the weight slowly, resisting all the way down until your arms are nearly straight.

**Concentration Curls**

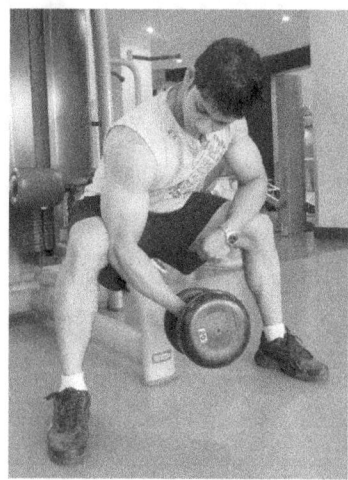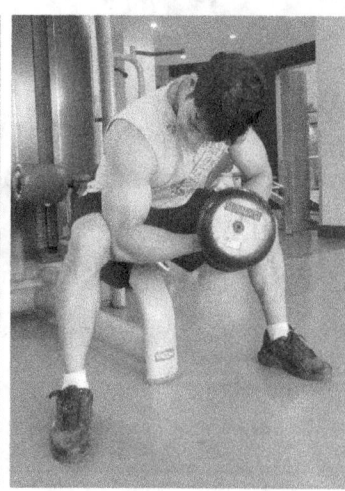

Sit on the end of a flat bench. Spread your legs apart into a V and lean forward slightly. Grasp a dumbbell in one hand with your palm facing upward. Rest your elbow on the inside of your thigh and let the dumbbell hang. Rest your other hand on the top of your other thigh for support. Slowly curl the weight up while keeping the torso, upper arm and elbow still. As you lift, twist your wrist so that your little finger turns towards your body. Squeeze the muscle at the top and then slowly lower the weight.

## Preacher Curls

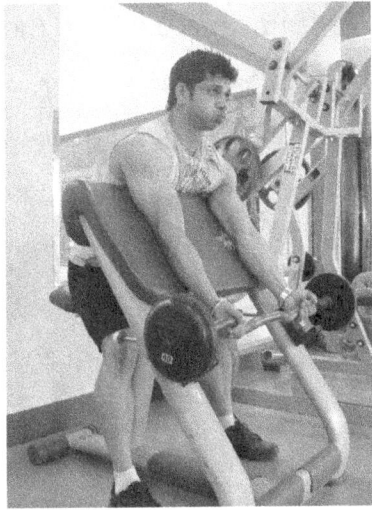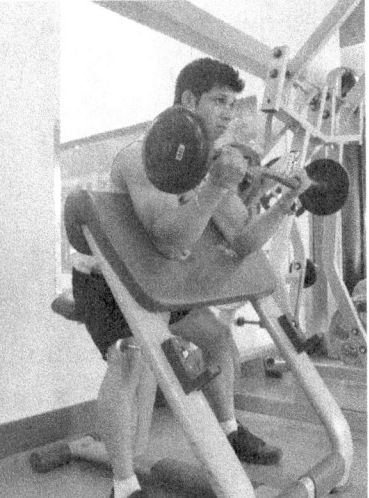

Using a preacher curl bench and an EZ curl bar, make sure the seat is adjusted to the correct height. The seat should not be so low that the shoulders are elevated nor so high that you're hunched over the pad. Grasp the bar using a shoulder width grip. Curl the bar upward in an arc. Curl the bar towards your chin, but keep in mind that the resistance is greater at the beginning of the rep. Go down slowly and work the muscle on the way down.

## Hammer Curls

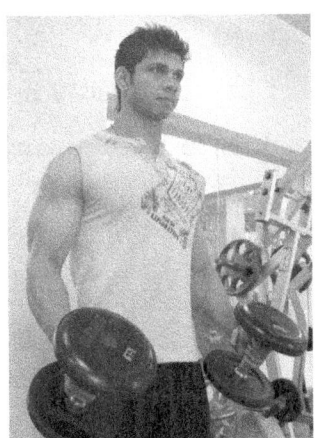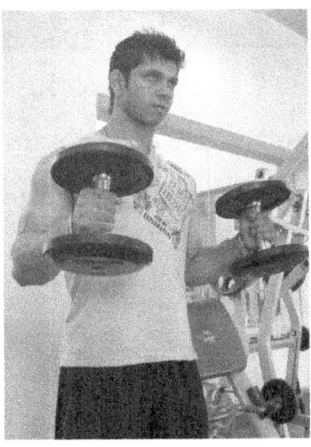

With a dumbbell in each hand, stand with your arms hanging at your sides, palms facing each other. Keep your elbows locked into your sides. Your upper body and elbows should remain in the same place during the entire exercise. Keeping your palms facing each other, curl the weight in your right hand up in a semi-circle toward your right shoulder. Squeeze the biceps hard at the top of the movement and then slowly lower. Do not turn your wrists during this lift. You can also do one arm at a time and/or alternate. Be sure to squeeze your biceps for a one-count at the top of the movement. Slowly lower the dumbbell to the start position and then repeat.

**E.Z Bar Curls**

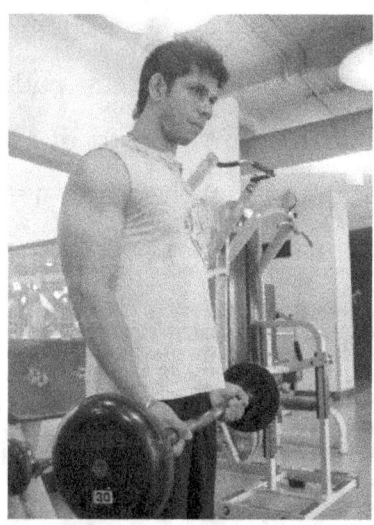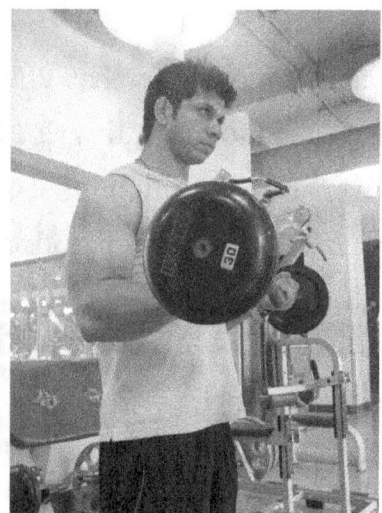

Just like a normal barbell curl, but with an EZ Curl bar. Position your hands so they are on the curve that allows your palms to face inward toward one another. To build higher peaks in the arms you should adopt a closer grip.

## Cable Curls - Wide/Close Grip

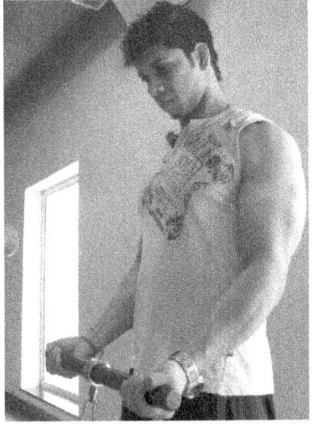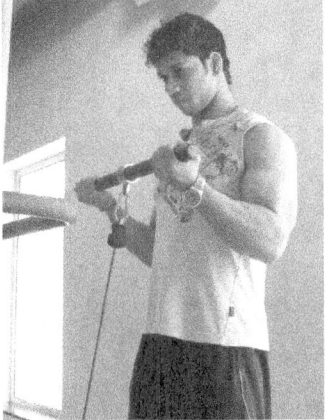

Stand facing a low pulley machine and grab a short bar attached to the low cable with an underhand grip (using both hands). Simply curl the bar up so as to try and touch it to your shoulders. Keep your elbows locked firmly in place at your sides throughout the movement. Slowly return to the start position and repeat.

## Lying Straight Bar Cable Curls

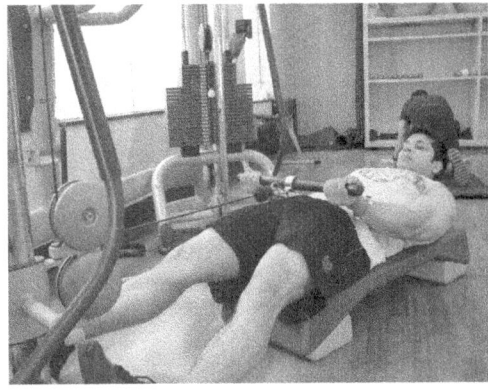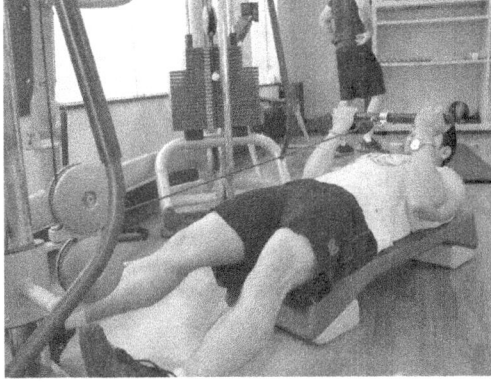

Lie flat on your back in front of the low-pulley weight stack with your feet flat against the frame of the machine, keeping your legs straight. Grab a cable bar and attach it to the machine, using an underhand grip. Rest the bar on your thighs and slightly bend your arms. Slowly curl the bar up toward your chest, squeezing your biceps for a one-count.

## Cable Rope Hammer Curls

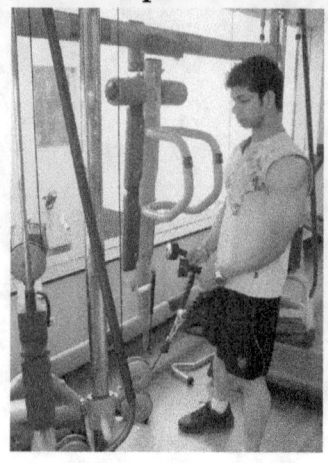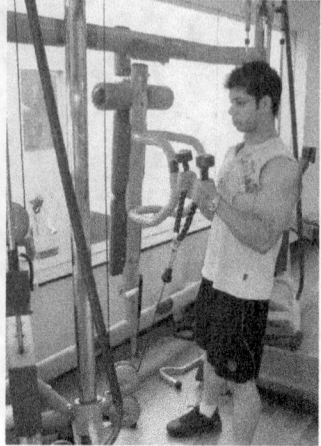

Use a rope attachment fixed to the low pulley machine. Grab the rope with your palms facing in toward your body and stand straight up. Put your elbows at your side and keep them locked there. Curl your arms up so as to have your hands try and touch your shoulders, keeping your wrists locked and your palms remaining facing inward.

## Chin-Ups

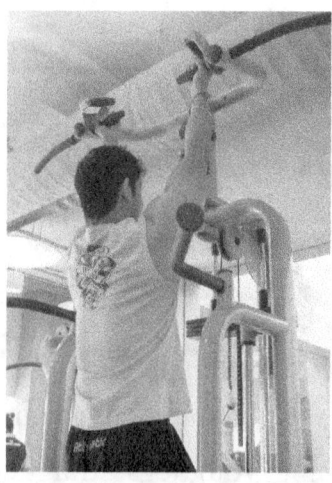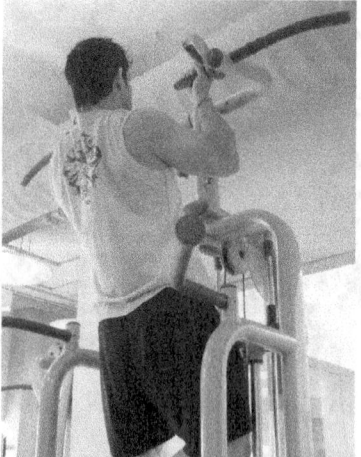

Grab the chin-up bar with a reverse grip and your hands just beyond shoulder-width apart. Pull yourself up and try to touch either your chin or upper chest to the bar. Return slowly to the starting position and repeat until failure.

# **Forearm** Exercises

Optional Exercises which can be incorporated on a separate day or with your bicep workout.

**Barbell Wrist Curls**

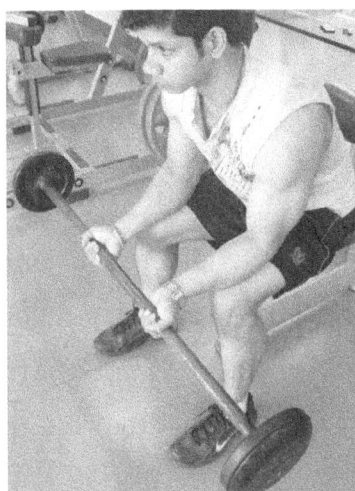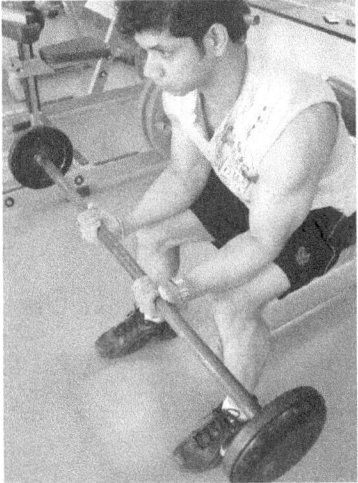

Hold a barbell with both hands and your palms facing up. Your hands should be about 16 inches apart. Sit at the end of a bench with your feet flat on the floor and about 20 inches apart. Lean forward and place your forearms on your upper thighs and the back of your wrists over your knees. Lower the bar as far as possible, keeping a tight grip. Curl the bar up as high as possible. Do not let your forearms move! Can also be performed with two dumbbells.

## Reverse Barbell Curls

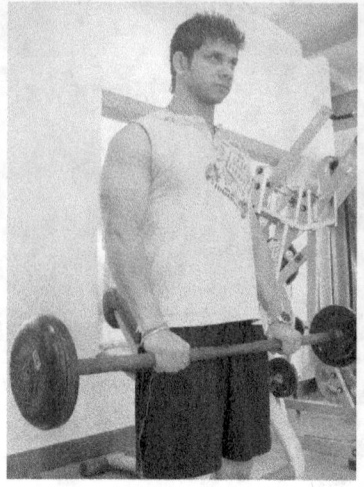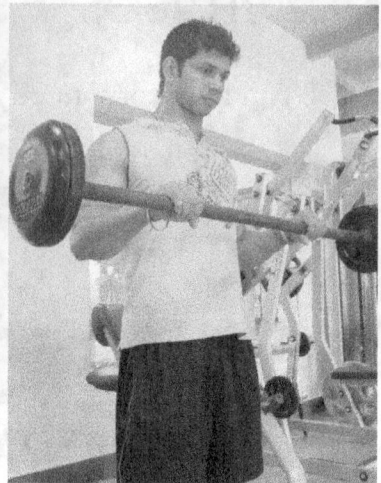

Grab a barbell and stand with your feet about shoulder width apart. Let both arms hang down in front of your body, fully extended with your palms facing in toward your body. Next, lift the barbell upward, similar to a Hammer curl. Slowly return to the start position and repeat. Be sure to keep your elbows locked at your sides throughout the entire movement.

## Wrist Curls Behind the Back

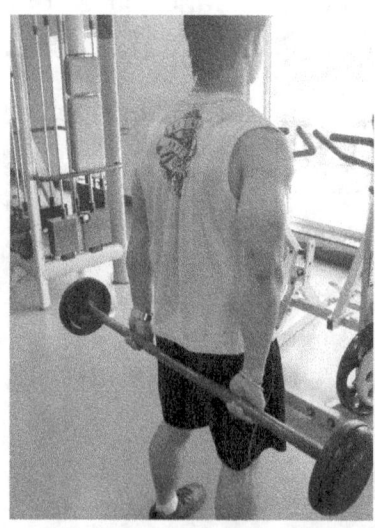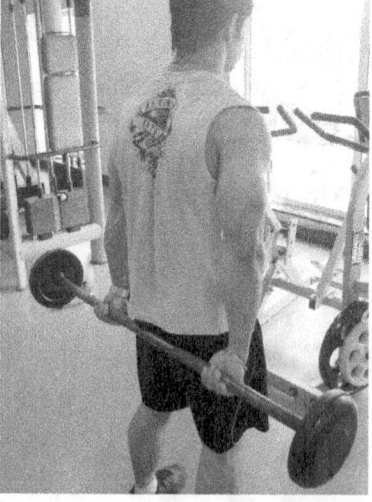

While standing with your feet about shoulder width apart, grab a barbell with both hands using an overhand grip, but with your hands and the barbell behind your back. Curl the barbell up toward the ceiling using only your wrists and forearms. When returning to the start position, allow the bar to roll into your fingertips and then repeat.

**Reverse Cable Curls**

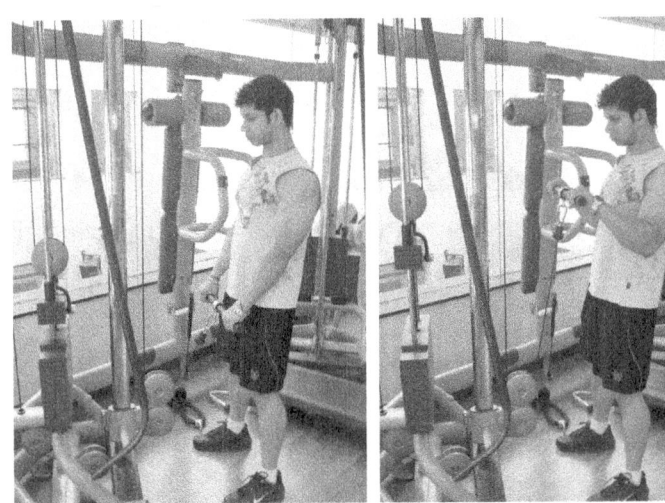

This exercise is similar to the reverse barbell curl exercise except that you will be using a short bar attached to a pulley machine. Stand with your feet about shoulder width apart and grab a short bar attached to a pulley machine with both hands, palms down. Begin with your arms hanging down, fully extended. Curl the bar up to a level that is parallel to the floor. Be sure to keep your elbows locked in place throughout the movement and to focus on having your forearms do the work.

# **Shoulder** Exercises

### Dumbbell Shoulder Press

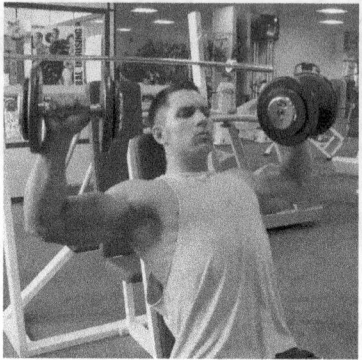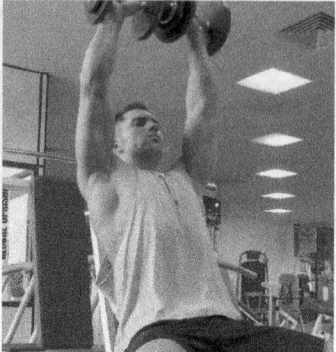

Position yourself on a bench or chair with your back upright and straight. Grasp a dumbbell in each hand and hold them just outside of each shoulder with your thumbs pointing in toward each other. Simply press the dumbbells up over your head and return to the start position just outside your shoulders. Repeat this movement for the desired amount of repetitions.

### Front Raises

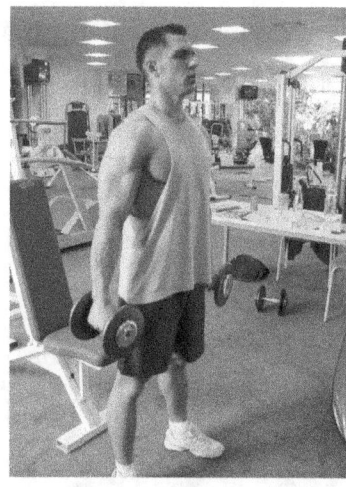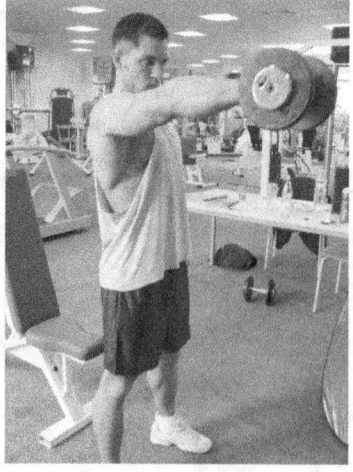

Stand with your feet about shoulder width apart. Hold a dumbbell in each hand letting your arms hang straight down and your thumbs facing in toward one another. Simultaneously raise one the dumbbells upward to where your arms become parallel to the ground. Pause for a one-count at the top of the movement and then slowly return to the start position and repeat.

**Side Raises**

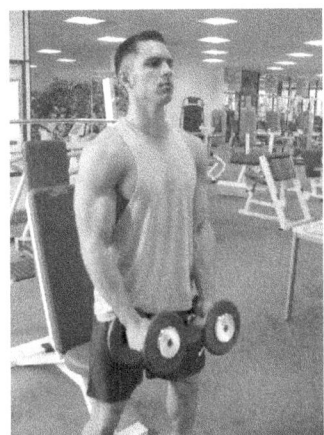 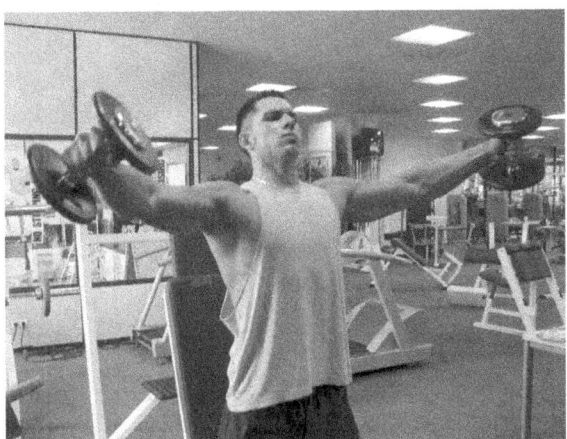

Stand with your feet approximately shoulder width apart and grasp a dumbbell in each hand allowing the dumbbells to hang down at your sides with your palm facing in toward your body. Next, simultaneously raise the dumbbells by bringing the backs of your hands to the ceiling, keeping your arms as straight as possible throughout the movement. Bring your arms to a point that is parallel to the floor, hold for a one-count and return to the start position and repeat for the desired repetitions.

**Upright Row**

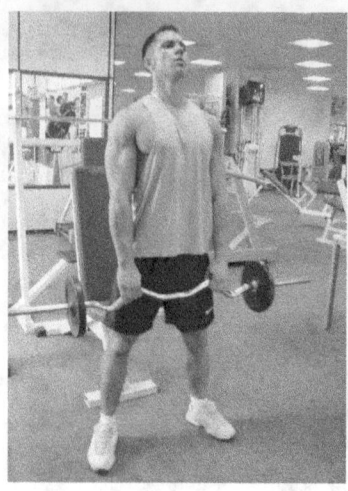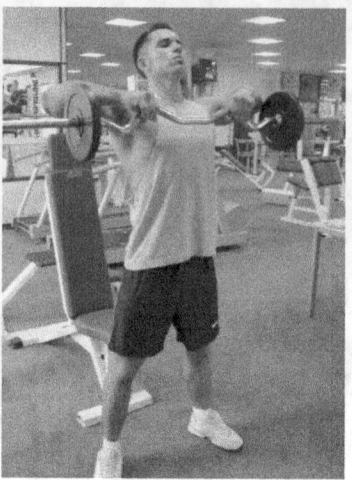

Stand with your feet approximately shoulder width apart. Using a narrow overhand grip, grasp an EZ Curl Bar or Straight Bar with both hands and let the bar and your arms hang down in front of your body, fully extended. Next, raise the bar up to just under your chin. You will do this by flaring your elbows up and out.

**Side Cable Raises**

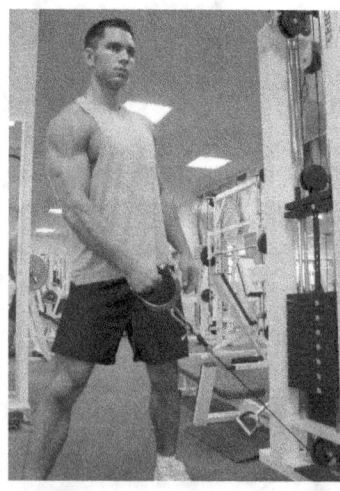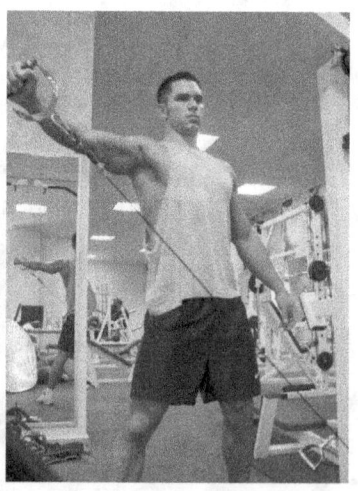

Attach a single handle to a cable pulley and adjust the settings so that the pulley is at its lowest position. Stand with the side of your body approximately two feet from the cable pulley. Take a small step back so that the cable can run across the front of your body when the exercise is being performed. Grab the single handle with the hand furthest away from the cable pulley. Stand with your back straight and feet shoulder-width apart. Bend slightly at the elbow and raise your arm to the side until it is level with shoulder height. Squeeze for a count of one and lower your arm toward the starting position. However, before your arm is directly at your side (about an inch away), raise your arm for the next repetition.

# **Trap** Exercises

Optional Exercises which can be incorporated on a separate day or with your shoulder or back workout.

### **Dumbbell Shrugs (Traps)**

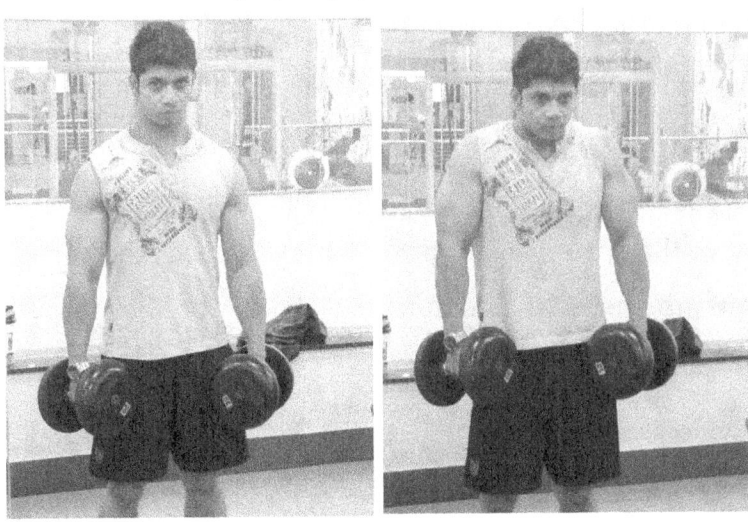

Stand with your legs about shoulder width apart and hold a dumbbell in each hand with your palms facing in toward your body. Allow the dumbbells to hang at your sides so that your arms are fully extended. To execute this movement, simply shrug your shoulders while keeping your arms completely straight. Be sure that you hold your shoulders in the shrug position for a one-count at the top of the movement. Return to the start position and repeat for the desired amount of repetitions.

**Cable Shrugs (Traps)**

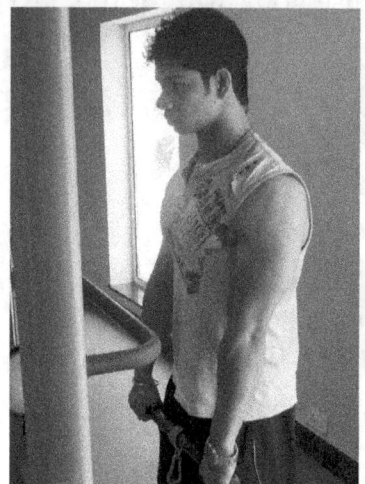 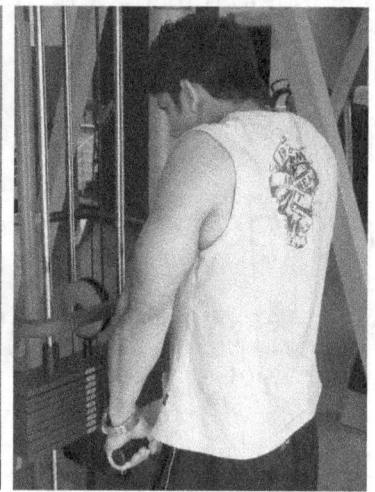

Stand facing a cable pulley machine with your feet about shoulder width apart. Attach a short bar to the low cable pulley. Grasp the short bar with both hands using an overhand grip and allow your arms to hang down completely straight. To execute this movement, simply shrug your shoulders while keeping your arms completely straight. Be sure that you hold your shoulders in the shrug position for a one-count at the top of the movement. Return to the start position and repeat for the desired amount of repetitions.

## Barbell Shrugs (Traps)

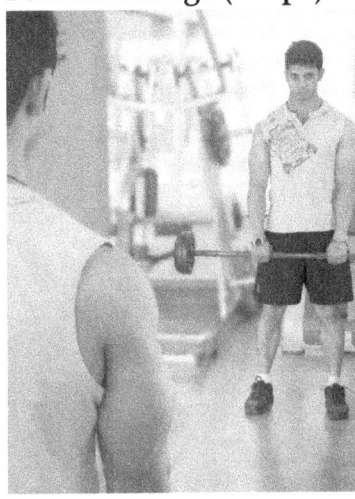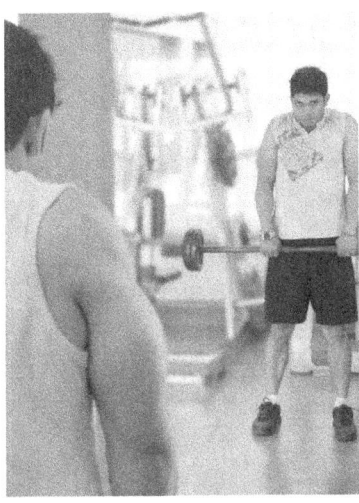

Stand with your legs about shoulder width apart and hold a barbell with both hands. Using an overhand grip, allow the barbell to hang down in front of your body so that your arms are fully extended. To execute this movement, simply shrug your shoulders while keeping your arms completely straight. Be sure that you hold your shoulders in the shrug position for a one-count at the top of the movement. Return to the start position and repeat for the desired amount of repetitions.

## Hand Grips

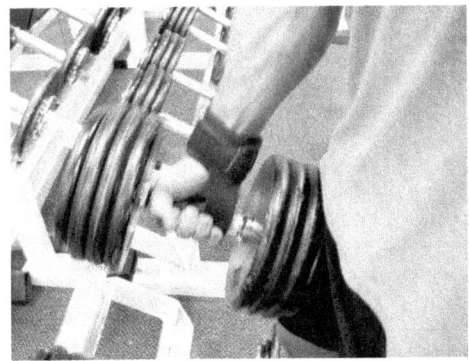

As you progress with the program I would suggest investing in some lifting straps. Straps are perfect for Lat Pulldowns, Shrugs, Deadlifts or any movement, set or exercise requiring a sure grip.

# **Tricep** Exercises

**Close Grip Bench Press**

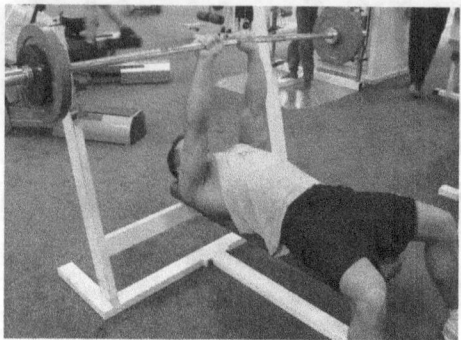 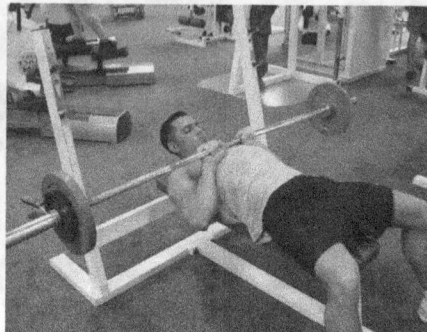

Positioning yourself on a flat bench. Lie flat on your back and grab the barbell above you with a very narrow grip. Focus on keeping a 6-8 inch width in your grip. Lift the barbell off of the rack and slowly lower it to about 3 inches above your chest and then press the bar back to the start position. Make sure to focus on keeping your elbows in towards your body throughout the full range of the movement.

**Dumbbell Kickbacks**

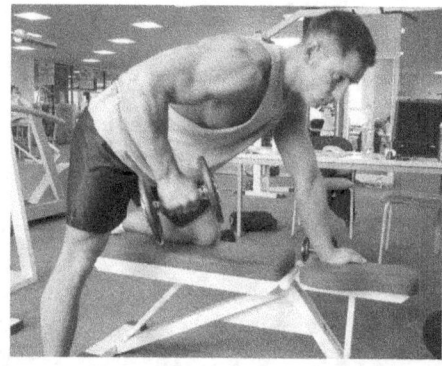 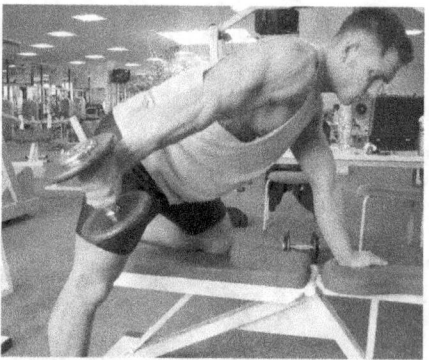

With a dumbbell in your right hand, position your left knee and hand onto a flat bench as shown. Keep your arm tucked into your side. Extend your arm out keeping your elbow in. At full extension of the movement, make sure to keep a little bend in your arm and all the tension on your tricep muscle. Then, slowly lower the dumbbell back to the starting position. Repeat with your opposite arm.

**Tricep Extension**

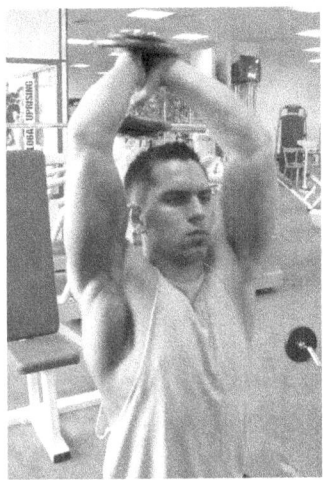 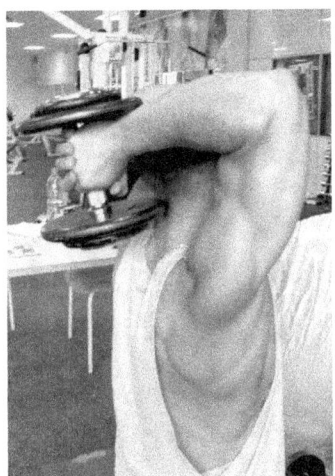

Sit on a low-backed chair or bench and lift a dumbbell over your head, holding it with both hands, palms cupped together. Keep your upper arms in place next to your head. In a slow continuous motion, lower the dumbbell behind your head. Feel the stretch in your triceps and then, using an equally slow and controlled motion, press the weight back up to full extension.

**Straight Bar Pushdowns**

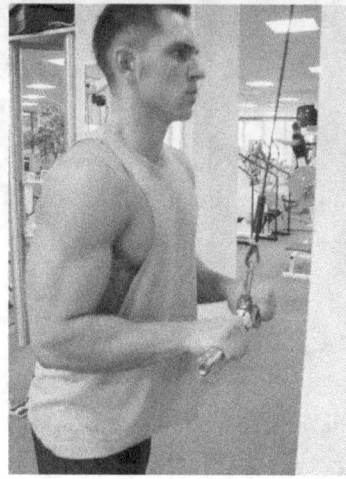 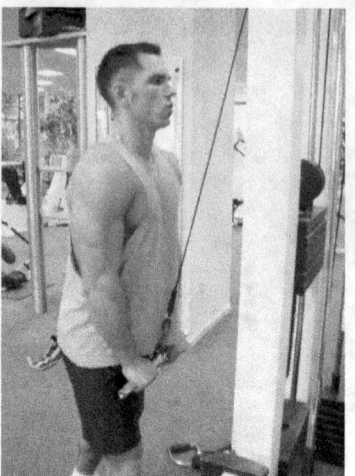

Attaching a straight bar to the top portion of a cable machine. Grab the bar with your palms facing down and position the bar at about chest level and then slowly lower the bar downwards. Be sure to keep your elbows in while extending your arms and have a slight bend in them when you reach the bottom. Slowly let the bar come back up to the starting position while keeping your elbows in.

**Cable Extensions**

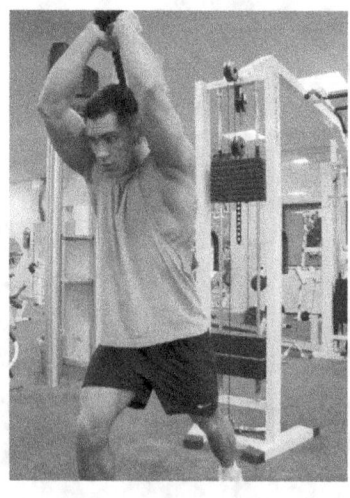 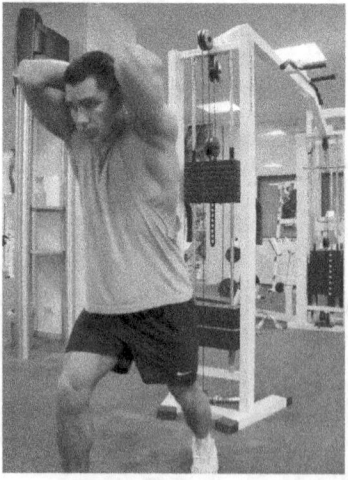

Using a rope attachment on the lower part of a cable machine, position your body away from the rope so your back is facing it. The best way is to have someone hand you the rope attachment in this position. Firmly grasp the rope attachment with your palms facing together and position the rope directly behind your head with your elbows in. Slowly extend the rope upwards, keeping your elbows in. Keep a slight bend in your arms when you reach the top position to make sure you keep the tension on your triceps muscle and off your elbow joints. Slowly lower your arms back into the starting position while keeping your elbow is throughout the range of the movement.

## Cable Extensions Alternative

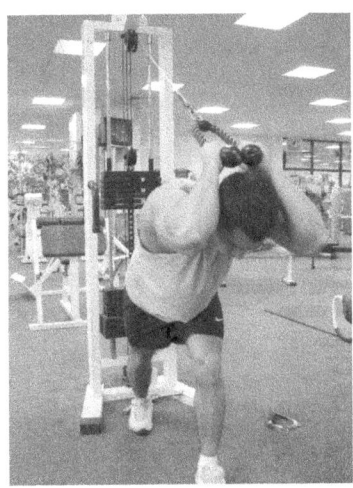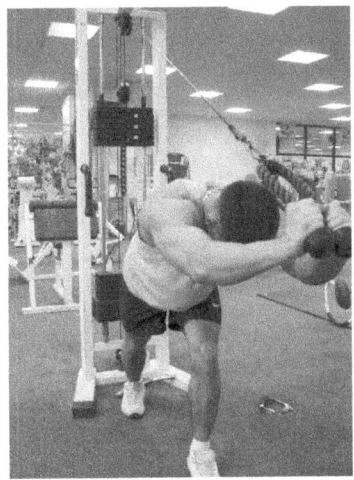

Using the same approach as above but with the the rope attachment placed on the higher pulley and your body positioned so that your upper body is almost parallel to the ground.

## Skull Crushers

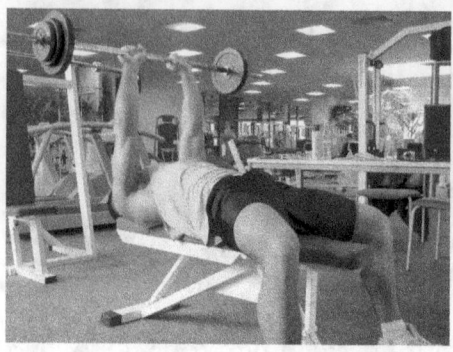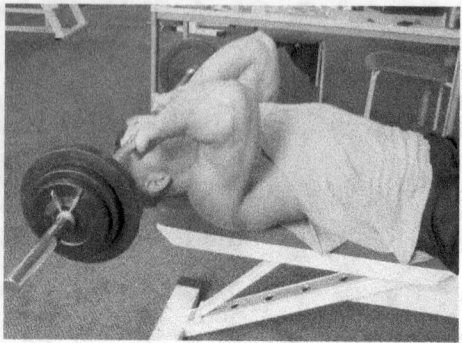

Laying flat on your back on a bench, grasp a barbell with your palms facing up. Hold the barbell tightly with your hands a few inches from your head. Extend your arms upwards, keeping your elbows in. Be sure to keep a little bend in your arms and all the tension on the tricep muscles. Slowly lower the weight back to the starting position while keeping your elbows in during the entire movement. You can also use the EZ Bar with this exercise.

## E.Z Bar Close Grip Press

Same as Close Grip Bench Press on page 146 but with EZ Bar.

# **Leg** Exercises (Quads)

**Leg Extension**

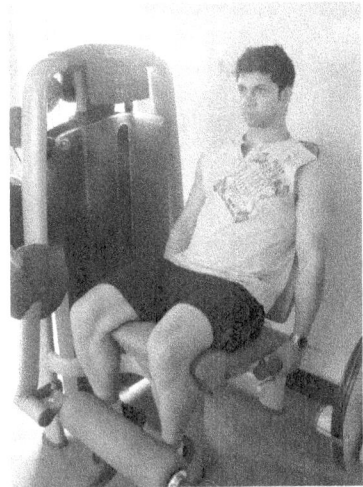 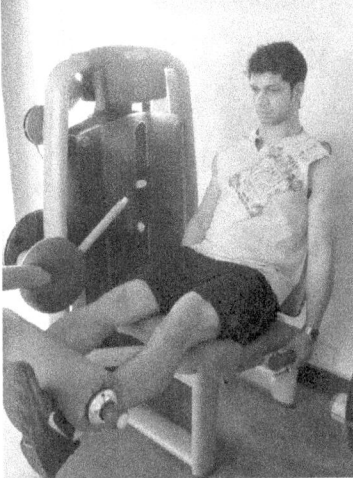

Position yourself in a leg extension machine. Begin by lifting the weight by extending both legs out and up, flexing at the knees. Lighter weight will produce more definition in the legs and help to produce a more prominent tear drop effect at the bottom of your quadriceps. Remember, to squeeze hard at the top of the movement.

**Smith Machine Squats**

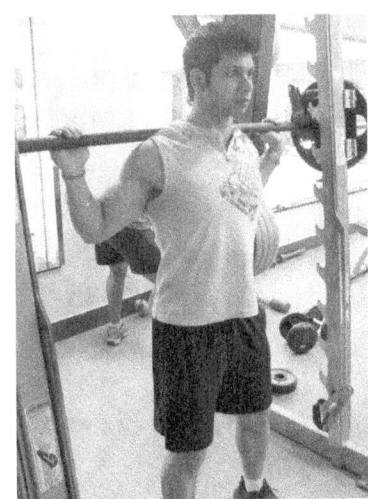 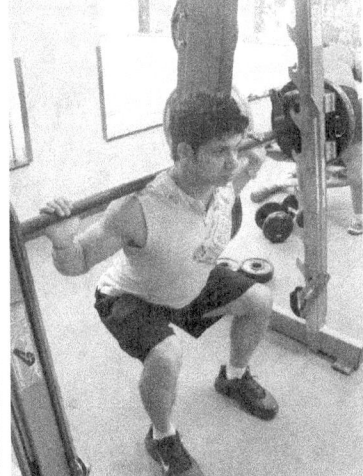

Using a Smith Machine, place the barbell across your shoulders behind your neck. Your legs should be a bit wider than shoulder width apart. To execute this exercise properly, simply squat down until your thighs become parallel to the floor. Visualize sitting down into a chair and be sure that you keep you back as straight and upright as possible throughout the entire movement. Return to the start position and repeat.

**Lunges**

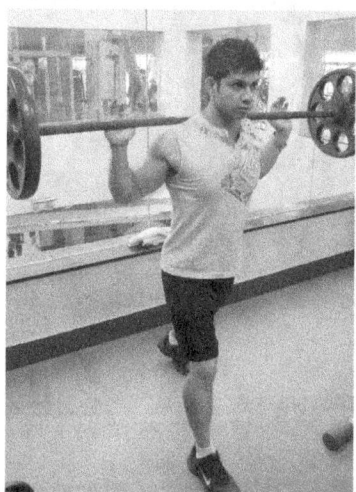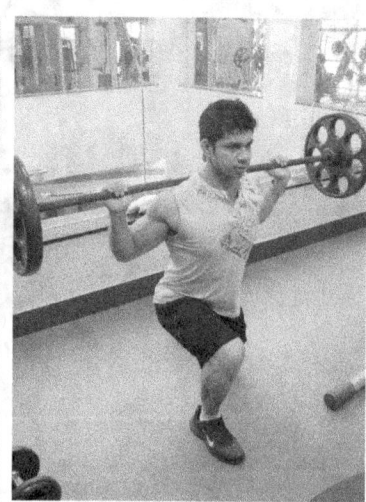

Place a barbell behind your neck and rest it across your shoulders. Be sure that you have enough room to perform this exercise. Begin by striding forward with one leg to execute a regular lunge while keeping the other leg set in place. Be sure to really stride forward so that you get a great stretch. Bring that leg back to the start position and repeat with the opposite leg.

## Leg Press

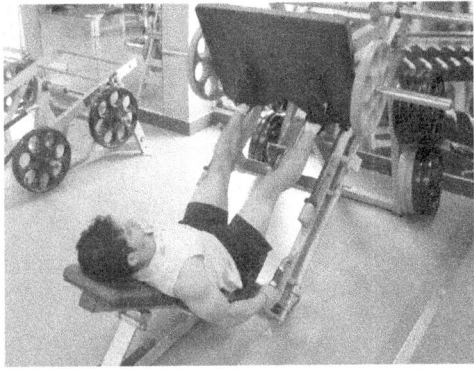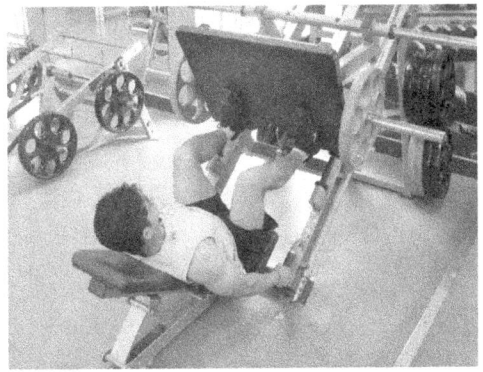

Position yourself in the Leg Press Machine with your feet about 12 – 15 inches apart. Slowly bring your knees in toward your chest, lowering the weight platform. Once lowered, return the platform to the start position by fully extending your legs (however, do not lock your knees out- allow there to be a slight flex at the top of the movement). This exercise can also be performed one legged to place more stress on the quads.

## Free Squats

Place a barbell behind your neck and securely rest it on your shoulders. Your feet should be just beyond shoulder width apart. Begin this exercise by squatting as though you are going to sit down in a chair. Squat to a point to where your thighs become parallel to the floor and then return to the start position. It is very important that you keep your back as straight as possible throughout 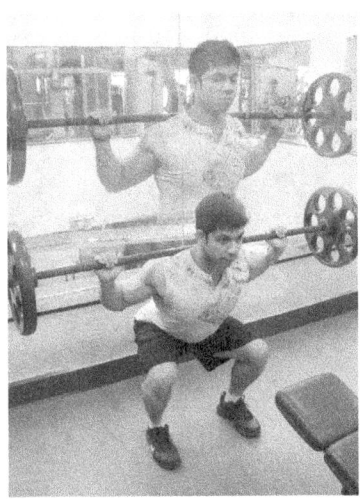 this movement, one way to help do this is to focus your eyes straight ahead during the entire exercise.

# **Hamstring** Exercises

### Standing/Seated Hamstring Curls

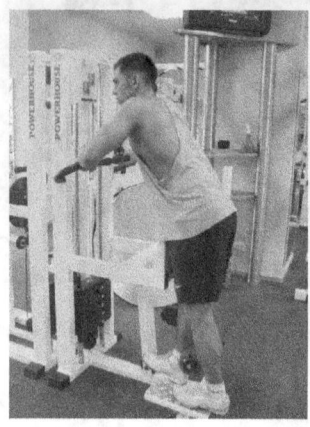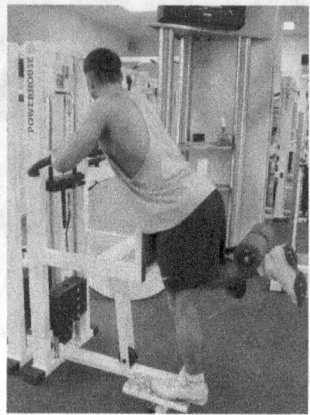

This exercise is also known as standing leg curls. Using the hamstring machine begin by curling the weight upward so as to touch your heels to your butt. As an alternative, shown below is the seated machine. Your gym may have a lying curl machine which can also be used.

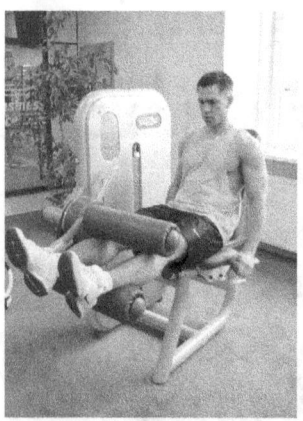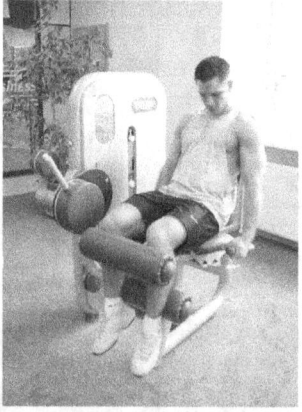

# **Calf** Exercises

### Barbell Calf Raises

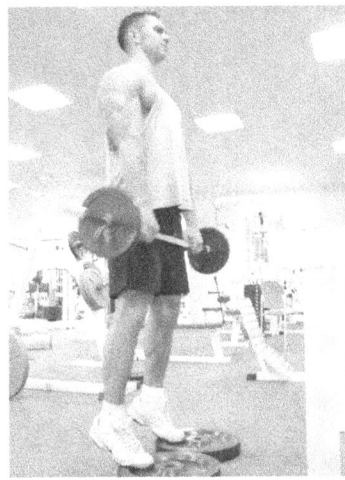 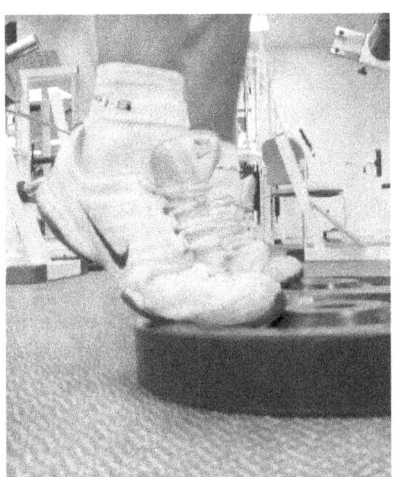

Stand in an area near a squat rack and place a barbell in your hands (you may add weight plates to the barbell for added resistance). This movement is similar to the seated calf raises. You may either position your toes over a weight plate or block of wood. Begin by pushing your toes down so that your heels become raised so that you are on your tip toes. Be sure to really flex your calves at the top of this movement for a one-count. [Can also be performed with dumbbells]

### Leg Press Machine Calf Press

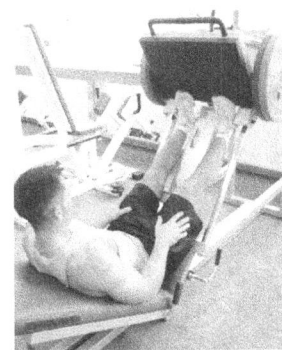 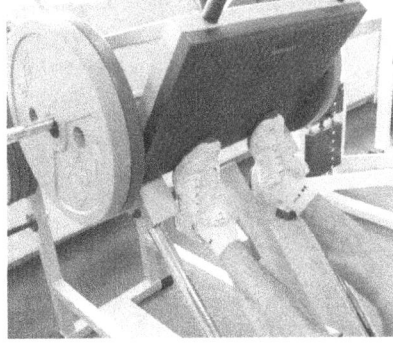

Using a leg press machine, position yourself as you normally would in the seat. Place your toes on the lower edge of the platform. Begin the exercise by pushing the platform forward/up with your toes (you can add weights to the platform for added resistance). Be sure to hold the platform at the top of the movement for a one-count and return to the start position and repeat until failure.

**Calf Machine Raises**

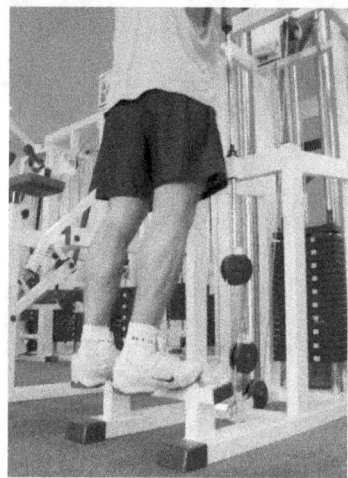 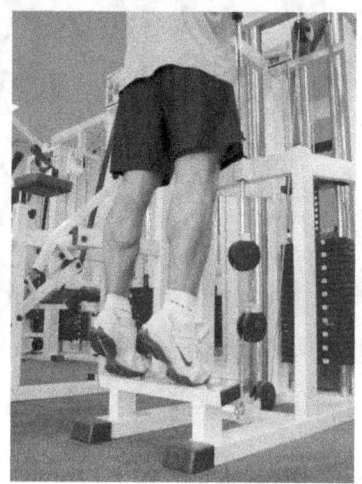

Stand on a calf raise machine. Under control, lower the weight from your ankle joints. Stop before you are all the way to the bottom and push the weight directly back up. Pause at the top, then reverse the motion back down.

# **Back** Exercises

## Lat Pulldown

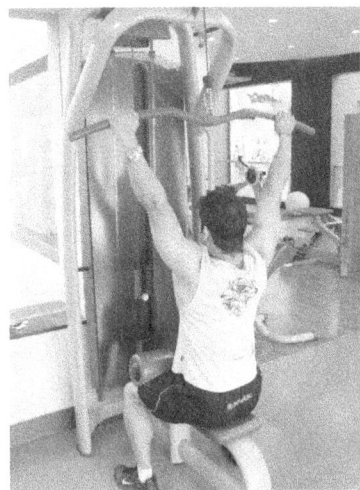 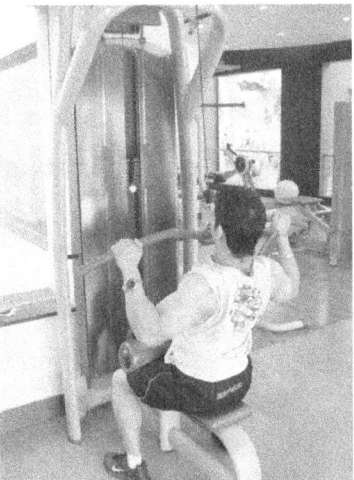

Position yourself on the lat pulldown machine and grab the bar with an overhand grip with your hands as wide apart as possible. Next, simply pull the bar straight down in front of you until it is about even with the middle of your chest. Slowly return the weight to the start position.

## Wide Grip Pull Ups

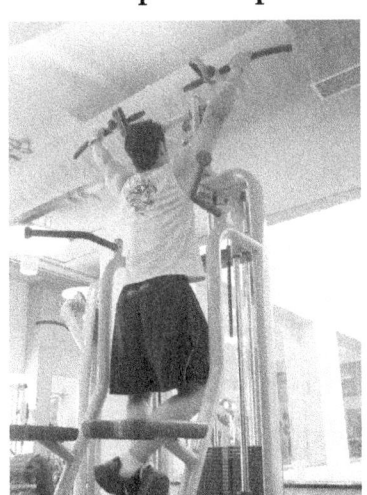 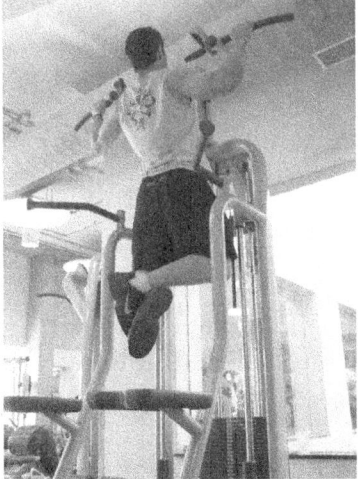

Find a pullup bar and grab the bar with your hands as wide apart as comfortably possible using and overhand grip. Next, simply pull your body up as high as possible so as to try and touch the back of you neck to the pullup bar. Slowly return to the start position and repeat.

### Close Grip Pulldown

Same as Lat Pulldown, but using a V-Bar attachment for a narrower grip.

# **Middle Back** Exercises

### Barbell Rows

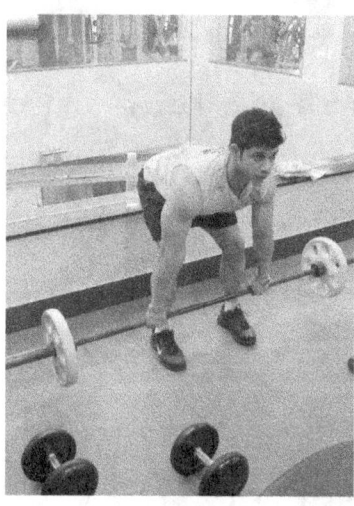 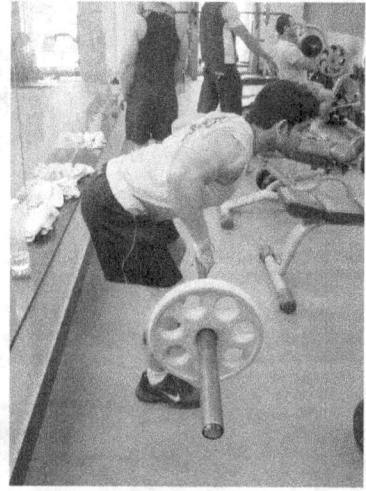

Grab a barbell and get in an area where you have a good amount of room. Bend forward at your waist so that your chest is leaning forward over your feet. Keep your knees slightly bent and your feet just beyond shoulder width apart. Grasp the barbell with both hands, using an overhand grip and having your hands about shoulder width apart. Start with your arms fully extended, allowing the barbell to hang at about mid-shin level. Next, lift or 'row' the barbell up and into your stomach area. Be sure to keep your head up and shoulders back throughout this exercise to keep your back in a firm and stable position.

**Two Arm Dumbbell Rows**

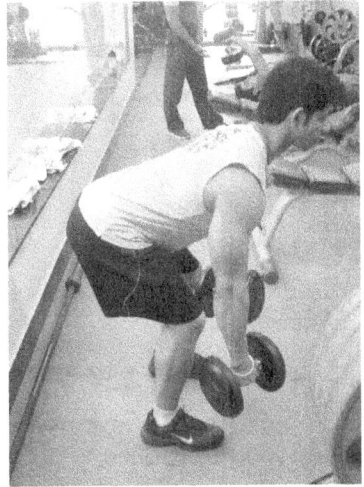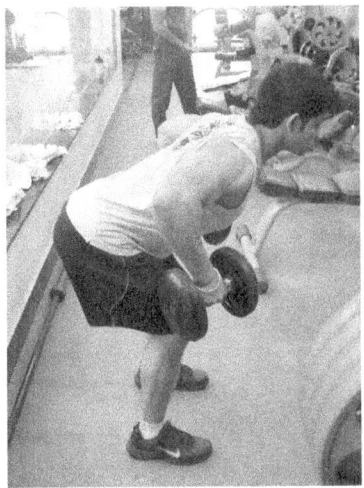

Grab a dumbbell in each hand and get in an area where you have a good amount of room. Bend forward at your waist so that your chest is leaning forward over your feet. Keep your knees slightly bent and your feet just beyond shoulder width apart. Start with your arms fully extended, allowing the dumbbells to hang straight down at about mid-shin level. Hold the dumbbells so that your thumbs point in toward one another. Next, lift or 'row' the dumbbells up and into your stomach area. Return to the start position and repeat. Be sure to keep your head up and shoulders back throughout this exercise to keep your back in a firm and stable position.

## Reverse Grip Barbell Rows

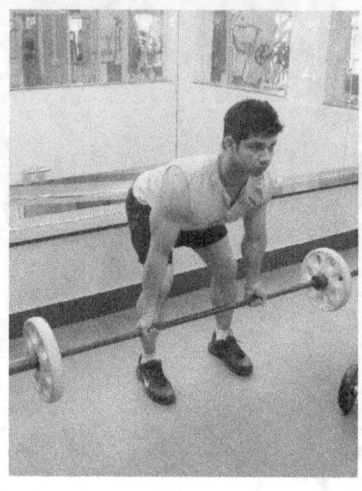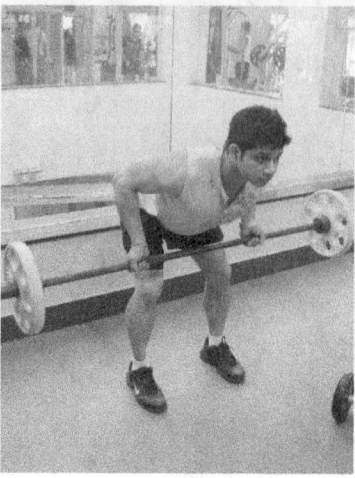

Grab a barbell and bend forward at your waist so that your chest is leaning forward over your feet. Keep your knees bent and your feet shoulder width apart. Grasp the barbell with both hands, using an underhand grip and having your hands about shoulder width apart. Start with your arms fully extended, allowing the barbell to hang at about mid-shin level. Next, lift or 'row' the barbell up and into your stomach area. Be sure to keep your head up and shoulders back throughout this exercise to keep your back in a firm and stable position.

## V-Bar Cable Rows

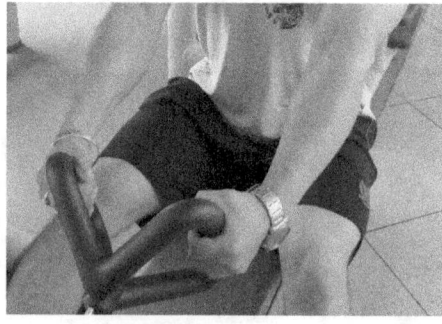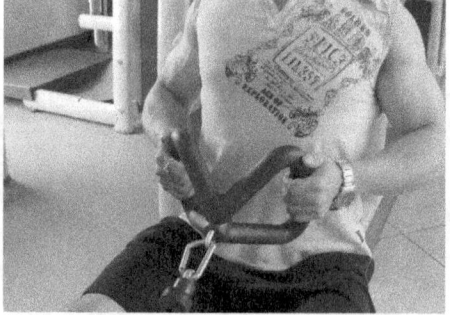

Performed exactly as shown on next page but using the V-Bar attachment.

## Cable Rope Rows

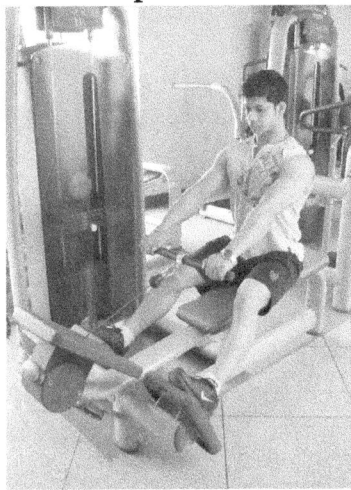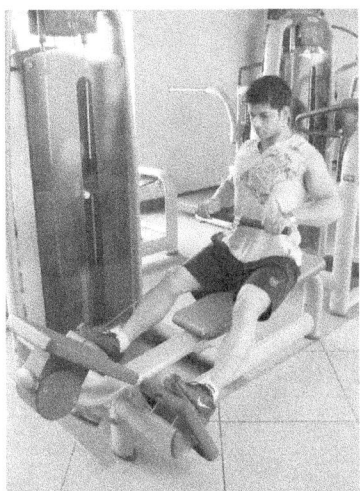

Attach a cable rope or single hand attachments as shown to a low-pulley cable and sit on a flat bench facing the weight stack. Adjust the seat or your position so that when you place your feet against the footplate, your legs are slightly bent and your trunk is erect. Lean forward at your hips to grasp the rope handle with a pronated grip (palms facing the floor), then lean back until your torso is once again erect and your arms are straight. This is the start position. Inhale and hold your breath as you pull the rope toward your midsection while keeping your elbows near your sides. As your elbows approach your body, turn your palms downward so your grip is pronated. Pull your elbows as far behind your body as possible. Hold the peak contraction for 1-2 seconds, exhale and return to the start position. Keep your torso erect throughout the movement. Allow your arms to stretch and your shoulder blades to relax before repeating for reps.

**One Arm Rows**

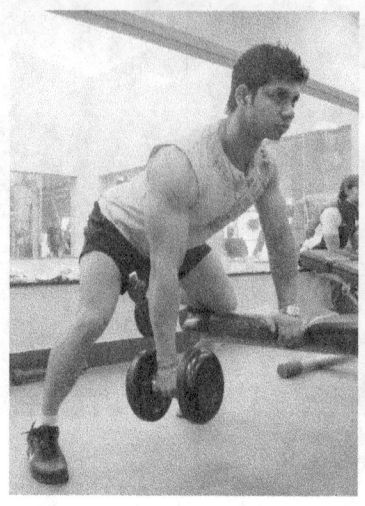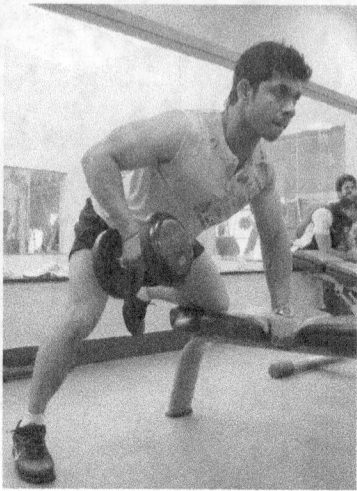

Place your left knee and left hand on a flat bench with your right leg set firmly on the floor. Lean forward so that your back is flat and parallel to the floor. Grasp a dumbbell in your right hand with your palm facing in toward your body and lift or 'row' the dumbbell up and into your outer rib cage area. Return to the start position and repeat.

## **Lower Back** Exercises

**Hyperextensions**

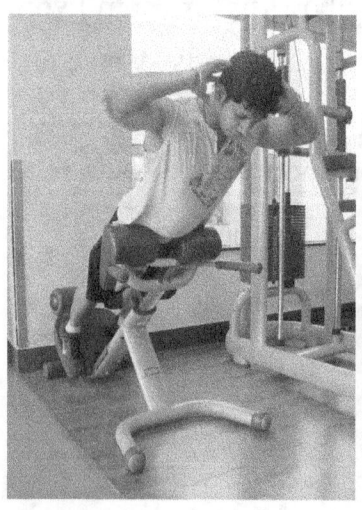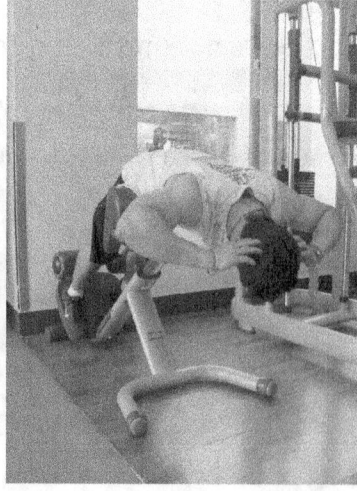

Position yourself on a Roman Chair facing forward. Cross your arms in front of your chest and slowly lower your upper torso down so as to try and touch your nose to the floor. Once your torso is completely bent over and virtually perpendicular to the floor, slowly return to the start position and repeat. Be sure that when you return to the start position that you do not arch your back at the top.

**Deadlifts**

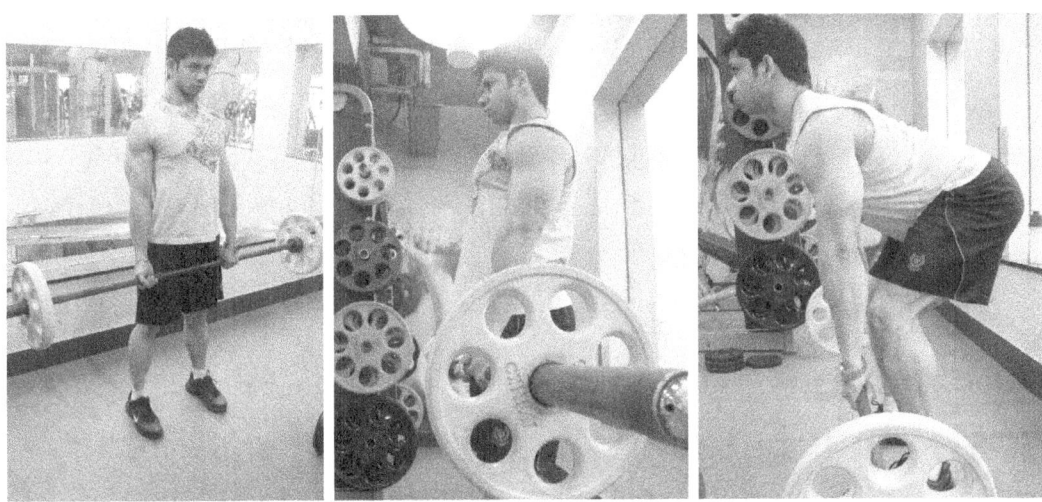

Grab the barbell with both hands using an overhand grip about shoulder width apart and let the barbell hang down in front of your body. Begin this movement by bending at the waist and lowering the barbell to the floor. Be sure to keep your legs as straight as possible (a slight bend is ok) and really let the weight of the barbell bring you down. On the way up, really focus on your butt and hamstrings to pull the weight back up. It is very important to keep your back straight and rigid throughout this exercise and to let your legs and butt do the work.

# ISOMETRIC STRETCHING

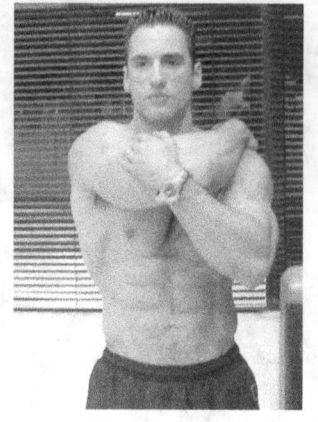

During a weight-training session, what do you do between sets? If you are like most people-you relax, talk to friends or maybe even check out a member of the opposite sex! While these activities might help you to waste the time, they do little to improve your physique. You should realize that your time in the gym is precious. If you really want to maximize your genetic potential, your actions must be dedicated to making optimal use of every training moment.

One of the best ways to make productive use of your rest intervals is to utilize a method called selective muscular stretching. Although many people regard stretching only as a means to increase flexibility, it can provide a multitude of muscular benefits when incorporated into your routine. In fact stretching a pumped muscle can enhance the quality of your workouts and help to promote muscular growth. Let's take a look at the benefits afforded by this practical technique.

### Reduced lactic acid build up

Nothing sabotages a workout more than the build up of lactic acid in your muscles. Lactic acid is a waste by-product of glycogen, a primary source of energy used to fuel your muscles during anaerobic exercise (weight-training). It's responsible for the burning sensation that accompanies intense training and eventually prevents your ability to achieve a muscular contraction. In simple words, once it builds up you simply cannot train any longer. Stretching helps to neutralize the negative effects of lactic acid by restoring blood flow to your working muscles. It provides an outlet to flush metabolic waste from your body, affording rapid regeneration of your muscular capacity.

**Better muscular recovery**

Contrary to popular belief, muscle tissue is actually broken down, not built up during a weight training session. This kind of damage contributes to the presence of delayed-onset muscle soreness that often accompanies a gruelling workout. However, by adapting stretching exercises you can repair muscle tissue and accelerate the healing process. The result is better recuperation between workouts, allowing you to come back strong for your next training session.

**Increased range of motion**

During weight training concentric repetitions cause your muscle to shorten. Over time they can adapt to this reduced length, restricting their range of motion. This limitation decreases the amount of force you are able to generate in your contractions and therefore compromising any muscular gains. Stretching exercises help to counteract these adverse effects, elongating your muscles to pre-exercise levels. You maintain greater elasticity in your joints and connective tissue, facilitating your ability to work though a full range of motions. Moreover, since your body is more flexible, you are less likely to exceed its stress barriers, reducing the possibility of an unpleasant injury.

As a rule stretching should be static. For example you slowly work into each stretch in a controlled fusion. Static stretching is the most effective method to achieve optimal benefits without potential damage to your muscular system. It allows for a gradual elongation of muscle tissue, permitting you to safely stretch your body to its utmost degree. For best results stretching should be included into your workout regimen on a regular basis. As soon as a set is completed, immediately stretch the muscle being trained by utilizing the movements discussed below. Try to hold each stretch throughout the entire rest interval and then proceed directly to your next set.

**Here's how:**

**Chest Stretch** - From a standing position grasp any stationary object such as a pole or exercise machine with your right hand. Your arm should be straight and roughly parallel with the ground. Slowly turn your body away from the object, allowing your arm to go as far behind 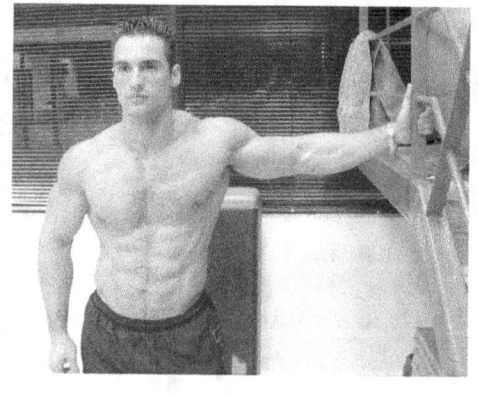 your body as comfortably possible. Hold this position for the desired amount of time and repeat the process on the left. Use this exercise during your chest workout.

**Shoulder Stretch** - From a standing position grasp your right wrist with your left hand. Without turning your body, slowly pull your right arm across your torso as far as comfortably possible. Hold this position for the desired amount of time and repeat the process on the left. Use this exercise during your shoulder workout.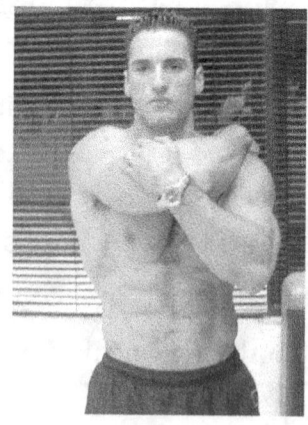

**Lat Stretch** - From a standing position grasp any stationary object such as a pole or exercise machine with both hands. Bend your knees and sit back so that arms are fully extended and supporting your weight. Shift your weight to the right in order to isolate 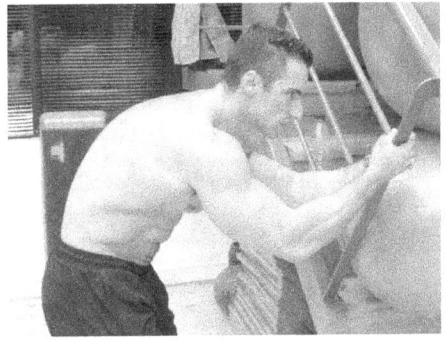 the right portion of your lathed this position for the desired amount of time and then shift your weight to the left. Use this exercise during your back workout.

**Triceps Stretch** - From a standing position raise your right arm over your head. Bend your elbow so that your right hand is behind your head. With your left hand grasp your right wrist and pull it back as far as comfortably possible, allowing your elbow to point toward the ceiling. Hold this position for the desired amount of time and repeat the process on the left. Use this exercise during your tricep workout.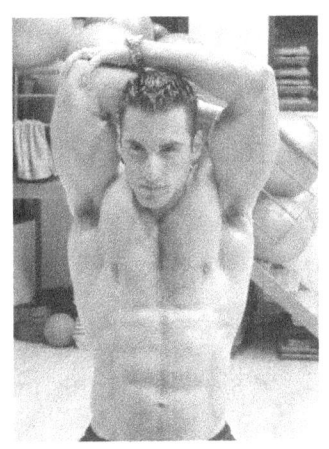

**Biceps Stretch** - From a standing position extend your right arm forward with your palm facing up. Place your left palm underneath your right elbow. Slowly straighten your right arm as much as comfortably possible, pressing your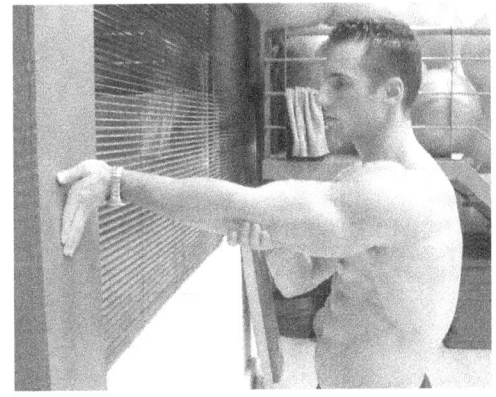

elbow down into your left hand. Hold this position for the desired amount of time and repeat the process on the left. Use this exercise during your bicep workout.

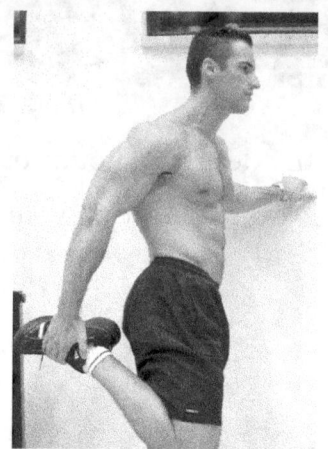

**Quadriceps Stretch** - From a standing position grasp a stationary object with your left hand. Bend your right knee and bring your right foot toward your glutes. Grasp your right ankle with your right hand and slowly pull your foot upward as high as comfortably possible. Repeat this process on the left. Use this exercise during your leg workout.

**Glutes Stretch** - Lie on your back with one leg extended fully along the floor and the other leg bent to 90 degrees and elevated. Place the same side hand on the hamstrings of this leg, just above the knee and place the opposite hand on the shin, just below the knee. By contracting your abs and hip flexors, reach the knee of this leg as far as possible toward the opposite shoulder. Use pressure from both hands to extend this movement slightly. Pause for one to two seconds at the end of the movement. Relax repeat this process to the opposite side. Use this exercise during your leg workout.

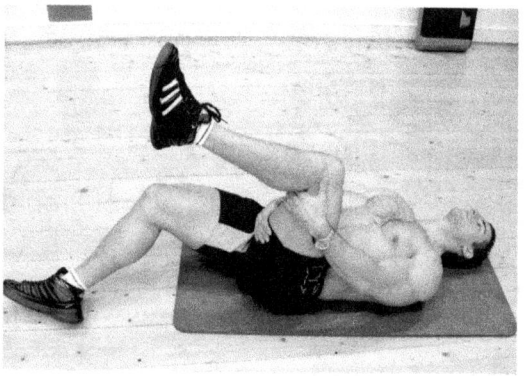

**Hamstring Stretch** - From a standing position straightens your legs and slowly bends forward at the waist. Allow your hands to travel downward along the line of your body as far as comfortably possible. At the point where you feel an intense stretch in your hamstrings, grab onto your legs and hold this position for the desired amount of time. Use this exercise during your hamstring exercise

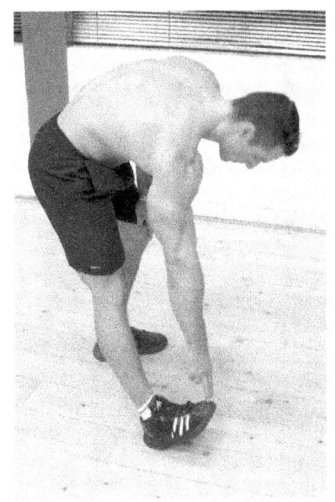

**Calf Stretch** - Stand on a raised block of wood or step and grasp a stationary object for balance. Take your left foot off the block so that you are standing on your right leg. Slowly allow your right heel to travel downward as far as comfortably possible. Hold this position for the desired amount of time and repeat the process on the left. Use this exercise with your calf exercises.

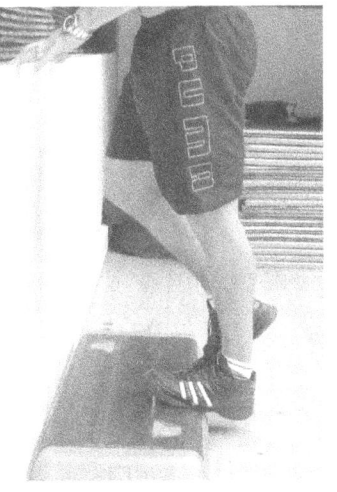

Undoubtedly stretching has various important benefits for a serious athlete because:

1) It aids dramatically in recovery by helping carry away a by-product of exercising metabolism, the lactic acid.

2) It prevents exercise injuries as it aids in the warm up process by helping deliver blood into the muscle.

3) It helps a lot with muscle separation. In other words if you are on a fat

loss diet and adapt stretching exercises you will look more cut than if you wouldn't do so.

4) It makes your muscular system well-developed and therefore you look bigger because of its muscle-lengthening capability

Other great forms of stretching include Yoga and Pilates. Although both are quite similar Pilates is designed to elongate, strengthen and restore the body to balance, whereas Yoga is really about creating balance in the body through developing both strength and flexibility. This is done through the performance of poses or postures, each of which has specific physical benefits.

# **NUTRITION** Continued

To reiterate what was explained earlier in the book, correct nutrition accounts for at least **80%** of lean muscle building success! You are what you eat - and this was never more true than it is for those wishing to change their physique. Before going into more detail I'd like you first to answer a few questions:

**Be honest with yourself**

- Do you often get depressed and irritable during the day or after workouts?
- Do you lack self-discipline or mental control?
- Do your workouts drain you so that it takes a sizeable amount of time to recover?
- Do you have difficulty maintaining enthusiasm for training?
- Do you suffer a great deal of muscular pain and burning?
- Do you suffer from constipation?
- Do you struggle to keep up energy levels during the day?
- Does your energy suddenly drain form you during workouts?
- Do you find no matter how much you eat and exercise you make little progress?
- Do you experience a lot of tiredness and fatigue?
- Do you find that when you put on weight it is fat and not muscle

If you've answered 'YES' to more than four of these questions then it is quite possible that your problems stem from **incorrect nutrition**.

This section will provide you with the essential facts on the nutrients that are vital for the Lean Muscle Success! and by applying the principles you can:

- Gain or lose weight according to your goals

- Increase lean muscle size

- Improve muscular structure and definition

- Maintain and increase energy

- Increase strength and stamina

- Keep your body cleansed, invigorated and stimulated

- Improve overall health

- Develop greater resistance to disease and sickness

- Gain an unbeatable edge on your friends

- Develop a superb physique!

Don't put off applying the principles you find here. The sooner you start, the sooner you will see results. And those results will introduce encouragement and enthusiasm that will add a powerful impetus to your training.

## THE MAIN NUTRIENTS

As outlined earlier in the book (Page 20) there are five main nutrients: Protein, Carbohydrates, Fats, Minerals and Vitamins.

### Protein

I touched on this earlier on, but in simple terms protein is the building block for muscle. Every single meal you consume from now on will contain some form of quality protein. Generally the best sources come from, chicken, turkey, fish, beef, egg whites, legumes, soy beans and whey/soy protein shakes and bars. Protein also contains essential amino acids, which work together to help you build leaner, stronger muscles.

Your body can only absorb protein in limited quantities at one-time (approx 50 grams), therefore a consumption of protein should be evenly spread out in every meal of the day (5-6 smaller sized meals). Not all protein is good protein for building muscle. It is also very important to possibly add a Whey/Soy Protein supplement which will provide not only good serving of protein, but all essential amino acids.

## Carbohydrates – The Energy Provider

Your body must have carbohydrates in sufficient quantities to be able to assimilate the protein. If your diet does not contain carbohydrates, your body will start using proteins for the purpose to provide energy - which means that protein will not be used to build muscle and tissue. Using protein for energy is also a slower process than using carbohydrates and you will be left feeling drained and often depressed and irritable. A low Carb/High Protein Diet is not the key here, but a Carb Rotation method will stimulate the very best results. More will be explained a little later in this chapter.

## Amino Acids

Proteins are made up of 22 amino acids which have to be present in certain combinations for the protein to function properly. If protein is to build and repair, it must have the right amino acids in proper quantities.

Without the right amino acids in the correct proportions, almost every physical process in your body will grind to a halt. In some cases, the amino acids need to combine with certain vitamins and minerals and if these are lacking, that particular body process will be impaired. Also a lack of amino acids to provide the right protein structure will make your body burn muscle for energy and store fat. If you find that you are eating and exercising a great deal and making no apparent progress your problem may lie here. This is why I strongly recommend a Whey Protein Supplement to use in conjunction with the program.

## CARBOHYDRATES Continued.

Carbohydrates supply energy. They are broken down to produce glucose (blood sugar) and stored in the muscle and liver as glycogen.

## Simple and Complex Carbs

Carbohydrates are divided into two main categories: simple carbohydrates and complex carbohydrates. Basically, the simple carbs provide quick energy and the complex carbs sustained energy. This type of Carbohydrate is generally found in processed foods like white breads, white rices, pizza, potato chips, candies and all snack foods.

**Note:** A predominance of simple carbohydrates in your diet will cause sharp fluctuations in blood glucose levels - and when that level suddenly drops - your energy levels take a dramatic dive. Recovery time after a workout will be longer and you will feel edgy and worn out. To make it simple avoid simple carbohydrates. Simple carbs add body fat!!

## Complex Carbs - The preferred Choice

The best sources of carbohydrates are 'Complex Carbs' and come from whole wheat and grain products, brown basmati rice, fruit, potatoes, vegetables, legumes and beans. Complex Carbs provide long lasting fuel for work and exercise, they will give you constant energy throughout the day.

The very best complex carb sources are: Whole Wheat Breads and Grains, Brown Rices, Shredded Wheat, Oats, Potatoes, Vegetables and Lentils.

Your pre-workout meals should all supply a serving of complex carbohydrates. Your last meal including complex carbs should be no later than 6pm, all meals after this time should be protein only with a fibrous carbs on the side (Any type of green vegetables are acceptable).

# A totally new approach to the
# **Low Carbohydrate Diet**

It's a fact that an intake of too many carbs will make you add body fat and too few will make you tired. So what is the answer? How can I lose body fat effectively while holding on to muscle?

Answer: **Carb Rotation**

For years, we were taught that carbohydrates were the food of choice for high energy and optimum athletic performance. We were taught that fat made us fat and carbohydrates made us lean and energized. Then everything seemed to change. Low carbohydrate diets have been with us for decades, but from the late nineties into the first few years of the new millennium, there has been a huge resurgence of interest in the low carbohydrate diet. Everywhere you look today there are low carbohydrate drinks, low carbohydrate meal replacements, low carbohydrate frozen dinners – even low carbohydrate pasta! Low carbohydrate dieting has definitely gone mainstream. Unfortunately, this has created a torrent of confusion and controversy. For every "guru" who says low carbohydrates are the ultimate fat burning diet, there is another "guru" with the opposite opinion. Who is right? Because of metabolic individuality, no single diet program is best for everyone. At certain times, for certain purposes, a low carbohydrate diet – done with a new approach you are about to learn - can accelerate fat loss beyond anything you've experienced before.

There are three secrets to getting all the benefits of a low carbohydrate lifestyle without all the side effects it might cause such as dramatic reduction in energy levels, changes in your mood and mental state, muscle tissue loss etc. The first is **carbohydrate tapering/manipulation**, which is the principle of eating more carbohydrates earlier in the day and fewer later in the day. The second secret is using **moderate carbohydrate reductions**, not the removal of all carbohydrates. The third is **carbohydrate cycling**. When combined, the results of these three techniques can increase fat loss beyond your wildest dreams and expectations! Let's take a closer look at each one.

## A) The carbohydrate tapering technique for maximum fat loss

If you want to get leaner quickly, a simple way to accelerate fat loss is to reduce the size of your late day meals. This technique is known as "calorie tapering" or "carbohydrate tapering." Simply cut out the starches (processed carbs) in your meals after 6pm, leaving the green fibrous carbohydrates, lean proteins and essential fats. Examples of late day fibrous carbohydrate and lean protein meals include; (1) Broccoli and Chicken Breast with a 1 tablespoon of flaxseed oil, (2) Tuna fish in a green salad with olive oil & vinegar dressing, (3) Asparagus and Salmon. (4) Egg White Omelette, (5) Low Fat Cottage Cheese with raspberries, (6) Whey or Casein Protein Shake, (7) Cuts of Chicken Breast in a Tikka or Chinese style sauce with green salad. When you drop the starchy carbohydrates (breads, cereals, desserts, potatoes etc.) from your last two meals, your ratios will automatically shift towards less carbohydrates and higher protein. It's an incredibly simple and easy technique to use, yet it can cause dramatic fat loss.

## How the low carbohydrate, high protein diet can benefit trainees

For very brief periods, athletes/fitness competitors often decrease their carbohydrates to only about 25% of their total calories. This is considered a "low carbohydrate" diet. This is the kind of diet a body-builder or physique competitor would use to prepare their physique for competition condition where fat levels need to be at there lowest. (This is why it's often called the 'pre-contest diet' see page 271). It can also be put to good use for any person looking to shed fat effectively.

### Pre-contest Diet:

Low carbohydrate, High protein

25-30% carbohydrates

50% protein

20-25% fat

For the average 150 pound male, this diet includes about 150 to 200 grams of carbohydrates per day. For the average 120 pound female, the carbohydrate intake is about 90 to 130 grams. This is just enough carbohydrates to stay alert and fuel high intensity workouts. A larger drop would be overkill. The protein intake is often very high for large and highly active individuals - as high as 300 grams per day for men and 175 to 200 grams for women. This usually works out to about 1.5 grams per pound of bodyweight. Most people except the world's best body-builders would argue that this is far too much protein, which it probably is if you stayed at this level all the time. However, if you reduce your carbohydrates to 25-30% of your total calories and you don't increase your protein and or fat to compensate, your calorie deficit will be too large. Whenever the calorie deficit is too big, you trigger the starvation mode. If you're uncomfortable with the idea of consuming this much protein, then you'll have to make up the difference in calories with essential fats, which in my opinion makes more sense (for example, 30% carbohydrate, 30% fat, 40% protein). Keep in mind that these extremely high protein levels are temporary and are usually maintained for only 12 weeks prior to a physique contest. Afterwards, you would gradually shift back to a baseline diet with more carbohydrates and less protein for maintenance.

## Sample Low Carbohydrate Menu

## INDIAN EXAMPLE

Meal 1 – 7:00 am : Breakfast Chapatis with Egg Whites

Meal 2 – 9:30 am : Whey Protein Shake with 1 scoop of oats

Meal 3 – 12:30 pm : Chicken Korma with 1 Chapati

Meal 4 – 3:30 pm : Whey Protein Shake with 1 scoop of oats

Meal 5 – 6:00 pm : Tandoori Chicken Kebabs with Spinach Dhal

Meal 6 – 8:30 pm : Low Fat Cottage Cheese


## WESTERN EXAMPLE

Meal 1 – 7:00 am : Oatmeal, 2 scoops whey protein, handful of almonds

Meal 2 – 9:30 am : Bagel, egg white omelet with pepper, onion, tomato

Meal 3 – 12:30 pm : Small serving brown rice, top round steak, broccoli

Meal 4 – 3:30 pm : Whey Protein Shake or MRP, wholegrain bagel

Meal 5 – 6:00 pm : Salmon, asparagus, 1 tablespoon of flaxseed oil

Meal 6 – 8:30 pm : Green salad, olive oil & vinegar dressing, tuna fish

This menu also uses the carbohydrate tapering method, only in this case, the starchy carbohydrates are cut off after 3:30pm. Meals one through four are protein and starchy carbohydrate meals, while meals five and six contain only lean proteins and fibrous carbohydrates. In addition, the serving sizes of the starchy carbohydrates in the first four meals has been reduced. Healthy fats are consumed in 3-4 meals, but can be split amongst all six if preferred.

### B) Carbohydrate "Cycling"

A low to moderate carbohydrate and high protein diet will cause much faster fat loss than a high carbohydrate diet. However, it may seem like the disadvantages outweigh the benefits. Fortunately, there's a solution to these problems and it's called "carbohydrate cycling." or "carb rotation". Some people refer to carbohydrate cycling as "zig zag" dieting, "Hi-low" dieting, "carbing-up" or carbohydrate "re-feeding." Regardless of what you name it, carbohydrate cycling is probably the **most powerful fat burning strategy on the planet**. Nothing else even comes close! It is the only guaranteed way to overcome the body's starvation response when calories and carbohydrates are low. Not only do you avoid a negative response, but you also invoke many positive responses that do not occur when holding your carbohydrates and calories at the same level day in, day out. That's the main problem with conventional low carbohydrate diets – they suggest that you drop your carbohydrates and keep them low. What I am suggesting is that you drop your carbohydrates according to your activity levels. We all know that carbohydrates are the source of your bodies energy supply. Eating too much causes fat gain, easting less causes fat loss! Therefore you need to rotate your carbs according to the days you exercise or are more active.

Days that you need carbs (and I'm talking good quality complex carbs here, like: wholegrains, wheats, fruits, vegetables, lentils, legumes, salad, brown rice, basmati, potatoes, oats,, rice cakes etc.) are the days you will be weight training. These will become known as your **HIGH** **HIGH CARB DAYS**. The days that you will not be training or the days you may just be doing cardio alone will be known as your **LOW** **LOW CARB DAYS.** On either of these days you should begin to reduce your carbs after 6pm or 5 hours before bedtime and stick to protein foods with green veggies, salad or maybe some rice cakes. **Anything like chapatis, dosas, idli's this late are not recommended**. Again this is due to the carbs not being burned off this late at night. If you eat a meal at 8pm with a large amount of processed carbs that food will be turned to body fat overnight, it's that simple. Therefore, late night binge eating with breads, cereals, cookies or desserts will need to be eliminated. If you find you would like even greater fat loss you can begin limiting processed/starchy carbs earlier in the day.

Carbohydrate cycling has been a well-kept secret of body-builders and fitness models for decades, but anyone can use it to accelerate fat loss or break a plateau. The beauty of this method is that it allows you to get all the fat loss benefits of low carbohydrate dieting without the low carbohydrate side effects. Most important, it keeps your metabolism elevated and prevents you from going into starvation mode.

Now in order for the carb cycling to work with your plan you may need to adjust your training days to cater for the low carbs, so it would be advisable to start your three low days on a Friday or Saturday, that way you can carb load on a Monday for your workout. You would then have a high carb day on Monday, low on Tuesday, moderate on Wednesday, low on Thursday and high on Friday before repeating. Again, you can fine tune this yourself depending on your workout frequency, but you should not exceed three days of very low carbs in a row. Why?

After three days in a row on very low carbohydrates (less than 90g per day), your glycogen levels will be almost completely depleted. If you were to continue on low carbohydrates for a fourth day, fifth day, or beyond, you would notice your energy and training intensity begin to diminish. You would also notice that your muscles would "flatten out" and become softer. Your metabolic rate would begin to slow down and your thyroid gland would decrease its output of thyroid hormone. Basically, your diet would become less and less effective the longer you stayed on low carbohydrates beyond the three day period. Your body is so "smart," it simply makes changes in physiology and metabolism to compensate for the prolonged lack of carbohydrates (which it interprets as starvation). That's why you have to keep your body guessing, by throwing in a high carbohydrate day every fourth day.

**High Carb Days and Low Carb Days**

Carbohydrate cycling is based on the concept of rotating low carbohydrate days with high carbohydrate days instead of keeping carbohydrates low all the time. Every fourth day your glycogen levels are restored with a "carb load" or "high carb day", your energy stays up, your muscles fill out and tighten and your metabolic rate gets a dramatic boost. The high day also makes your entire diet easier to stick with because no matter how difficult it is to get through those three low days, you have a "high carb day" to look forward to. The "high carb day" also bypasses all the side effects. You get noticeably leaner with every three-day low carbohydrate cycle as your body dips deeply into stored body fat without the carbohydrates readily available for fuel. Surprisingly, you may even continue to get leaner even on the high carbohydrate days because of the boost in metabolic rate. Carbohydrate cycling also prevents your body from becoming inefficient at using carbohydrates for energy. When you cut your carbohydrates out for a long time, your body begins depending on fat for fuel and it learns how to use fat for fuel more efficiently. You often hear low carbohydrate diet proponents say that the low carbohydrate diet turns you into a "fat burner" while a high carbohydrate dieter turns you into a "sugar burner." This may be true, but there's a huge downside to staying on low carbohydrates all the time and becoming an exclusive "fat burner:" Your body becomes lazy and inefficient at burning carbohydrates. When you eat them again after a long absence, your body doesn't know what to do with them. This is one of the reasons you will simply blow up overnight and gain weight back the minute you re-introduce carbohydrates after a long absence. Unless you plan on never eating a carbohydrate ever again, you'd better think twice about long-term carbohydrate restriction. Low carbohydrate diets 24/7 are not lifestyle programs, unlike the Carb Rotation method which can be implemented into your daily life long term. What's the alternative? Carbohydrate load every fourth day. When you carbohydrate load a depleted muscle, the carbohydrates are quickly soaked up by the muscle on that day because the muscles are "hungry" for carbohydrates. By repeated cycles of depletion and re-loading, your muscles become extremely efficient at storing carbohydrates as muscle glycogen rather than partitioning them to body fat.

# Fine tuning the carbohydrate cycling method

As you get leaner and leaner, you may find that you lose weight too quickly on the 3:1 carbohydrate cycling plan. Furthermore, it's not a wise idea to lose more than 2.0-3.0 lbs of body weight per week. If you lose more than three pounds per week, you are much more likely to be losing lean muscle mass with the fat. If you lose lean mass or drop weight too quickly, you should adjust your high to low day ratio by increasing your carbohydrates (and calories) overall or by keeping your low days the same and adding more high days. If you train with weights four days a week, you'll have four HIGH CARB DAYS and three LOW CARB DAYS. You can do three low carbohydrate days followed by the four high carbohydrate days, just adjust according to the days you train. You can even throw in a couple of moderate carb days if you like, which would typically be done on days you may only train one body-part, e.g. your back. Taking two or three high days after three low days will not only help reduce muscle loss, it may allow you to gain small amounts of muscle as you lose body fat. It's very difficult to put down one single example of 3:1 carbohydrate cycling as I've described it here and have it apply to everyone. A little bit of experimentation and fine tuning will be necessary to discover what amount of carbohydrate works best for your high and low days. It's absolutely essential for these types of advanced diets to be customized. On average, women would consume about 100 grams of carbohydrates on low days and about 150-200 grams of carbohydrates on high days. Men would consume 125-150 grams of carbohydrates on low days and 200-300 grams of carbohydrates on high days. Here are examples of what "typical" high-low cycles would look like on a fat loss program for the average person 150 pound male and 120 pound female:

**Macronutrients:** 1g of Protein = 4 cal, 1g of Carbs = 4 cal, 1g of fat = 9 cal

**Men/1940 calories/ low carbs:**

Protein 45% = 700 calories = 175 g

Carbs 30% = 700 calories = 150-175 g

Fats 25% = 540 calories = 50 g


**Men/2360 calories/ high carbs**

Protein 35% = 800 calories = 200g

Carbs 45% = 1000-1200 calories = 250-300 g

Fats 20% = 360 calories = 40 g


**Women/1460 calories/ low carbs**

Protein 40% = 600 calories = 150 g

Carbs 35% = 500 calories = 125 g

Fats 25% = 360 calories = 40 g


**Women/1715 calories/ high carbs**

Protein 35% = 600 calories = 150 g

Carbs 45% = 800 calories = 200 g

Fats 20% = 315 calories = 35 g


On your low carbohydrate days, eat protein and starchy carbohydrates in your early day meals (meals one through four), then in your late day meals (meals five and six) eat protein with only fibrous carbohydrates like green vegetables and salad – no starchy carbohydrates! On your high days, you can eat starchy carbohydrates with five of your meals (and if you're going to have a "cheat day" do it on a high day). So that's it! These are some very powerful techniques, but remember; carbohydrate cutting taken to the extreme will do more harm than good. Never cut your carbohydrates out completely and never stay on low carbohydrates for a long period of time. It's usually not wise to go to extremes in anything and this is as true for dieting as with anything else in life: Moderation is the key. For the Carb Rotation method to be successful you need to be strict, this doesn't mean you need to count carbs exactly gram for gram, certainly not, but you do need to familiarize yourself with the **Carb Lists**. The idea is to just keep your intake low on non weight training/cardio days and increase consumption on weights days.

**So how many carbs should I eat?**

These are just averages and you will need to fine tune yourself. But the general rule of thumb in regard to macronutrients is the following:

**MEN**

**HIGH CARB DAYS**

**Protein** 1.0-1.5 g per pound of bodyweight, **Carbs** 1.5-2.0g per pound of bodyweight, **Fats** no more than 40g per day (75% or more should come from unsaturated fat)

**LOW CARB DAYS**

**Protein** 1.0-1.5 g per pound of bodyweight, **Carbs** 1.0-1.2g per pound of bodyweight, **Fats** no more than 50g per day (75% or more should come from unsaturated fat)

## WOMEN

### HIGH CARB DAYS

**Protein** 0.8-1.2 g per pound of bodyweight, **Carbs** 1.5g per pound of bodyweight, **Fats** no more than 30-40g per day (25g or more should come from unsaturated fat)

### LOW CARB DAYS

**Protein** 0.8-1.2 g per pound of bodyweight, **Carbs** 1.0-1.2g per pound of bodyweight, **Fats** no more than 30-40g per day (25g or more should come from un-saturated fat)

You can of course taper the figures on the previous page according to your own goals and measurement of progress.

Low Carb Days – can go as low as 0.5g - 0.8g per pound of bodyweight
Moderate Days (light exercise or light activity) – approx 1g
High Carb Days - approx 1-2g per pound of bodyweight

*There are 4 calories in 1 gram of carbohydrates

### USEFUL CARB LISTS

The protein content in these foods is minimal and will not count towards your daily protein requirements.

| Breakfast foods/Cereals | |
| --- | --- |
| 1 slice of Brown/Wholemeal/Rye/Wholewheat Bread | 12g |
| Wholemeal Chapati | 12g |
| Wheat Crackers – Thin x 4 | 8g |

| | |
|---|---:|
| All Bran Cereal Medium Bowl | 30g |
| Weetabix – 2 biscuits | 25g |
| Wheaties Cereal – Medium Bowl | 23g |
| Special K – Medium Bowl | 35g |
| All Bran – Medium Bowl (50g) | 30g |
| Bran Flakes - " " | 30g |
| Muesli - " " | 30g |
| Cheerios " " | 30g |
| Oatmeal " " | 35g |
| Corn Flakes " " | 30g |
| Corn Grits " " | 30g |
| Oats (50g) | 33g |
| Low Fat Yogurt (Small Yogurt) 4oz Plain | 20g |
| Low Fat Yogurt (Small Yogurt) 4oz Fruit | 23g |
| Freshly Squeezed Orange Juice (1 tall glass) | 15g |
| Pure Grape Juice (1 tall glass) | 26g |
| Cranberry Juice (1 tall glass) | 35g |

## Fruits

| | |
|---|---:|
| Banana (1 Medium) | 27g |
| Apple (1 medium) | 30g |
| Orange (1 medium) | 15g |
| Grapes (approx 20) | 20g |
| Pink Grapefruit (1 half) | 10g |
| White Grapefruit (1 half) | 12g |
| Apricots (3 medium sized) | 12g |

| | |
|---|---|
| Raspberries (approx 20) | 15g |
| Dried Apricots (approx 10 large) | 25g |
| Raisins (California – handful) | 12g |
| Prunes (5 large) | 30g |
| Strawberries (approx 10) | 12g |
| Plums (1 small) | 9g |
| Kiwi Fruit (1) | 11g |
| Honeydew Melon (1/4) | 12g |
| Watermelon (1/4) | 8g |
| Tangerine (1 medium sized) | 11g |
| Mango (1 medium sized) | 17g |
| Gala Melon (1/4) | 6g |
| Pear (1 medium sized) | 28g |
| Peach/Nectarine (1 medium sized) | 30g |

## Vegetables/Salads

| | |
|---|---|
| Carrots (1 medium raw) | 7g |
| Carrots (boiled – large spoonful) | 12g |
| Cauliflower (4 spears) | 10g |
| Broccoli (4 spears) | 20g |
| Green Beans (10 beans) | 12g |
| Asparagus (4 spears) | 8g |
| Cabbage (1 large spoonful) | 7g |
| Parsnips (1 medium parsnip) | 10g |
| Corn on the cob ( 1 large) 100g | 20g |
| Kale (1 cup) | 8g |

Okra (80g) — 4g

Mushrooms (5 large) — 10g

Onions (1 large) — 16g

Eggplant (1 large) — 6g

Zuccini (3 medium sized) — 8g

Turnips (5 small) — 8g

Bean Sprouts (large serving) 100g — 10g

Spinach Boiled (large serving) 100g — 1g

Squash/Swede  "      "     " — 2g

Celery 1 stalk — 1g

Lettuce 1 large leaf — 1g

Radish (4 small) — 4g

## Pastas/Rice/Potatoes

| | |
|---|---|
| Brown Rice (Cooked/Boiled) 100g cooked weight | 22g |
| Basmati Rice (Cooked/Boiled) 100g cooked weight | 22g |
| Wholegrain Rice "    "    " | 22g |
| Wholewheat Spaghetti "   "   " | 22g |
| Macaroni   "        "        " | 28g |
| Boiled Potatoes (5 medium sized) | 20g |
| Baked Potato (1 medium sized) | 30g |
| Roasted Potatoes (5 medium sized) | 25g |
| Instant Potato (5 heaped tablespoons) | 25g |
| Sweet Potato (1 large mashed) | 24g |
| Yam (1 medium) | 20g |
| Noodles (Stir Fry) 100g | 14g |

## Snacks/Others

| | |
|---|---|
| Ryvita/Crispbreads x1 | 8g |
| Graham Crackers x 2 | 11g |
| Rice Cake | 5g |
| Skimmed Milk 100ml | 3g |
| Soy Milk 100ml | 3g |

**And how much protein do I require?**

Between 1.0-1.5g per pound of bodyweight. Those looking to add good lean muscle size should aim for the latter (1.2-1.5g). Women should stick at 0.8-1.2g per pound of bodyweight, again, the latter (1.2g) if looking to add muscle.

**Here is a list of foods high in protein:**

PROTEIN VALUES – You only need count the protein values in the foods on the following pages. The foods listed have minimal carb values and therefore do not need to be counted towards your daily carb intake.

## Poultry

| | Protein | Fat |
|---|---|---|
| Chicken Breast without skin (100g cooked) | 25g | 0.8g |
| Turkey Breast without skin (100g cooked) | 25g | 0.8g |
| Turkey Breast Mince (100g cooked) | 24g | 0.8g |
| Low Sodium Deli Chicken Slices (2 slices) | 10g | 2g |
| Chicken Chunks (Canned – 1 tin) (100g) | 18g | 1g |
| Low Sodium Deli Turkey Slices (2 slices) | 10g | 1g |

## Fish/Seafood – (Can be baked, grilled or steamed)

| | | |
|---|---|---|
| Tinned Tuna (1 tin) in water (125g) | 35g | 1g |
| Tinned Tuna (1 tin) in oil/brine (100g) | 32g | 1.4g |
| Salmon Tinned (1 medium sized tin) (100g) | 18g | 5.9g |
| Fresh/Frozen Shrimp/Prawns (100g ) | 18g | 1g |
| Crabmeat (1 medium sized tin) (100g tin) | 14g | 0g |
| Sole/Flounder Baked (100g cooked) | 15g | 0g |
| Haddock (100g cooked) | 24g | 0.7g |
| Cod – Medium sized portion (100g cooked) | 20g | 1g |
| Baked Salmon (100g cooked) | 20g | 7g |
| Baked Tuna (100g cooked) | 22g | 0.7g |
| Baked Trout (100g cooked) | 21g | 6g |
| Monk Fish (100g cooked) | 25g | 1.2g |
| Halibut (100g cooked) | 20g | 2.5g |
| Sardines (3 medium sized) | 18g | 11g |
| Mackerel (100g) | 19g | 12g |

## Meats – Red meats should be consumed no more than 3 times weekly

| | | |
|---|---|---|
| Sirloin Steak (Lean 100g cooked) | 25g | 7.5g |
| Rump Steak (Lean 100g cooked) | 25g | 9g |
| Beef – Roast Rib (Lean 100g cooked) | 25g | 12g |
| Stewing Streak (approx 10 chunks) | 18g | 3.5g |
| Lean Steak Mince (100g portion) | 20g | 4g |
| Lamb Roasted (3 chops) | 18g | 7g |
| Beef Heart – Braised 3oz | 22g | 4.5g |
| Pork Chop – 1 medium sized (40 grams inc. bone) | 12g | 4g |

| | | |
|---|---|---|
| Pork Ribs (1 Rib 50g) | 12g | 7g |
| Bacon – 1 lean rasher (no fat) | 6g | 5g |
| Luncheon Meat – 2 slices | 3g | 3.5g |
| Thickly Sliced Ham – 60g - 2 slices | 17g | 5g |
| Cold Roast Beef – 2 slices | 15g | 3g |
| Cold Roast Pork – 2 slices | 11g | 1.5g |

## Others

| | | |
|---|---|---|
| Egg Whites (1 white) | 4g | 0g |
| Egg Yolk (Yellow Part) | 2g | 4.5g |
| Soy Beans – 100g | 15g | 7g |
| Tofu – 1 piece | 4g | 2.4g |
| Low Fat Cottage Cheese 100g | 15g | 1.5g |
| Dry Curd Cottage Cheese 100g | 18g | 0.3g |
| Protein Bar 30g | 20-30g | 3-6g |
| Whey Shake/100ml of skimmed milk – 1 scoop (30g) | 26g | 2g |
| Whey Shake/100ml of skimmed milk – 2 scoops (60g) | 52g | 4g |
| Whey Protein Shake/100ml of water – 2 scoops (60g) | 45g | 1.5g |
| Soy Protein Shake 1 scoop (30g) 100ml water | 20g | 1g |
| Soy Protein Shake 2 scoops (60g) 200ml water | 40g | 2g |
| Goat Protein 1 scoop (30g) in water 100ml | 18g | 1.2g |
| Hemp Protein 1 scoop (30g) in water 200ml | 14g | 2.5g |
| **100ml of skimmed milk** | **3.3g** | **1g** |
| **100ml of soy milk** | **3.3g** | **1.7g** |

## and fat?

You should aim to consume no more than **3g of saturated fat** per meal and a further **5-6g of unsaturated fat**. So a total of no more than 25g unsaturated fat per day on Training Days and then just slightly more on Non-Training Days, approximately 10g extra un-saturated fat throughout the day (See Page 23 for more on fats).

Let's take a look at the daily macronutrients for a 150 pound male:

**PROTEIN:** 150 x 1.2g of protein = 175g of protein required per day divided between 6 meals = 30g of protein in each meal.

**LOW CARBS:** 150 x 1.4g of carbs on low carb days(non training days) = 200g divided between 5 meals (last meal should have very few carbs) = 40g per meal

**HIGH CARBS:** 150 x 2g of carbs on training days = 300g divided between 5 meals = 50-60g per meal (last meal should have very few carbs)

**FATS:** 5 meals x 2-3g of saturated fat = 10-15g of saturated fat per day

5 meals x 5g of unsaturated fat = 25g of unsaturated fat [35g per day on Non-Training Days]

**Note:**

You should try to avoid all foods with artificial bleaching, coloring and preserving agents. Make sure you always read the wrapper or packaging of any foods before you consume them. You must go easy on 'fast foods' and 'junk foods'. The fat and simple carbohydrates contained in them will have a devastating effect on your progress. Allow yourself one treat meal a week, preferably on a 'High Carb' Day.

## FATS

Fats are a source of long term energy and since they contain vitamins A, D, E and K are vital for building lean muscle tissue. Fat provides more than twice as much potential energy as protein and carbohydrates, but if your intake is high, it will be stored as body fat and not used as energy since the body will first use carbs and protein to produce energy first. The body can store as much as 100,000 calories of energy in the form of fat, compared to 2,000 in the form of carbohydrates. The fat content of your diet must not exceed 25-30%. Fats are divided into two categories - saturated and unsaturated.

**Saturated fats,** are found in many Indian foods. They are present in animal products like lard, non-skimmed milk products, meat and egg yolks. They are also found in pizzas, hamburgers, snacks, candies and all other processed foods. Saturated fats should be kept as low as possible. Ideally, you should consume less than 3-4g per meal or no more than 20g per day.

**Unsaturated fats** are rapidly consumed and are found in oily fish such as salmon and fresh tuna, avocados, nuts and seeds, sunflower and olive oils, tofu etc. These fats are preferred and are considered **'Healthy Fats'.** In addition to saturated fats above, you can consume a further 25g of un-saturated fat per day.

Regular training on a diet moderate in carbohydrates, about 30-45%, with 35-45% protein and 20-25% fats will give your body a lean, hard appearance with good muscle separation and definition. You can spread your fat intake out between meals, e.g. 8g in one meal and 10g in another as long as you do not exceed the total daily allowances, which are no more than 20g of saturated fat per day between five meals and approximately 25g of un-saturated fat in 5 meals = 40-45g total fat per day. On Non-Training Days this can be increased to as much as 35g between 5 meals = 50g total fat per day.

This amount of fat seems quite high, won't intaking this much fat, make be fatter? This is about as true as saying eating chicken will make you grow a beak!! The science behind this is that due to the lower carbs, especially on Low Carb Days, the higher fats will become a primary source of energy. Although carbs will still be very much present, it will free up the protein and let it do its work of repair and growth and enable the carbs to replenish glycogen stores.

* I encourage supplementation of Omega 3 oils with this plan. These can be purchased from all good stores. Another excellent source of healthy fats are unsalted nuts (peanuts, cashew nuts, pecan nuts, brazil nuts, hazelnuts, walnuts, pine nuts and almonds which are great). A small amount of these added to your meals will help reach your daily un-saturated fat targets outlined above.

**5-6 SMALLER SIZED MEALS, NOT THREE LARGE ONES**
If you want to perform at the top, get strong, get lean, and look and feel great, then eating five to six small meals is a nutrition strategy that you must not overlook. This strategy has been used by athletes for many years and it's really caught on among active lifestyles over the past decade, especially so among people who simply want to improve their

health. So what are the benefits of this?

Eating 5-6 small meals a day boosts your body's basal metabolic rate (BMR). A higher basal metabolic rate means that your body's resting metabolism allows you to burn more fat, even while you are not exercising. By boosting your metabolism (BMR), you can be burning fat while driving your car and even while sleeping!

- Eating 5-6 small meals a day improves protein utilization and muscle growth.

- Eating 5-6 small meals a day reduces insulin levels. Insulin plays a very important role in fat metabolism by increasing the uptake of fat from the bloodstream and into body cells.

Surely I will be eating more? Not necessarily, because you are basically dividing your traditional three large meals by half; thus, the 5-6 meals contain the same total amount of food. However you can actually eat more and still lose body fat, as the increase in your metabolic rate from eating these smaller meals will still occur.

**Whey Protein Shakes - The perfect meal Replacement.**

Eating these smaller more frequent meals may not be possible for everyone, so those who may have restraints should supplement with a meal replacement or Whey Protein shake. These will provide you with a small sized meal in just one shake and are essential if unable to eat whole foods. I recommend supplementing with a Whey Protein shake mid morning and mid afternoon (for strict vegetarians, Soy or Hemp Protein is recommended instead), therefore you only need to account for four other meals. If you need to bounce up your carb intake you can either have a serving of carbs on the side or mix some oats in with your shake. Alternatively, you can get some Meal Replacement Shakes (MRP's) which contain both a serving of protein and complex carbohydrates.

**Out with the old, in with new**

I'm sure you are now fully aware that to get in the best shape possible you cannot afford to sit back and dig in to McDonald's, pizzas, ice cream, popcorn, candy, cakes and the like. You know that to be successful with the program things must change and this requires a little effort and dedication on your part. To make the changes you have to stand up to your cravings and say 'no'. Once you've turned the corner and waved goodbye to the bad foods you're well on your way to success. Once results are witnessed you'll see exactly why the right foods are the core factor of the Lean Muscle Plan. To begin with you should allow yourself a four hour window once a week where you can indulge in a little cheating and enjoy some of the foods you love, but be careful and don't over do it!

# SUMMARY:

- Beginner to exercise? Start light and gradually increase the poundages over the coming weeks.

- Remember the importance of nutrition. A great body needs a great diet! You cannot afford to forget this.

- Concentrate on proper form

- Take exercises to MMF (Momentary Muscular Failure) This will ensure you are hitting those muscles with 100% intensity.

- Always warm up your muscles with a few light exercises to start your session. This will get the blood pumping and will lessen the risk of injury.

- NUTRITION – CARB ROTATE. You must remember to stick to: 'High Days' - Days you weight train & 'Low Days' Days you do little activity or days you only do cardio.

- Don't forget the healthy fats. Adding a little olive oil, nuts and seeds to meals will help meet your daily requirements of un-saturated fat.

- Get a training partner to help you get the most out of your workouts.

- Use the planner sheets. An example follows on the next page.

- Visit the website. www.thedailyplate.com, here you can access macronutrient information for thousands and thousands of foods.

# High Carb Meal Planner Example

| | HIGH CARB DAY | Meals | | |
|---|---|---|---|---|
| 1 | | | | |
| 2 | | **Fats** | **Carbs** | **Protein** |
| 3 | **Monday** | 20% | 45% | 35% |
| 4 | Breakfast Chapati (2 wholewheat | | | |
| 5 | chapatis). 1 scoop of whey in water | 4 | 30 | 40 |
| 6 | | | | |
| 7 | | | | |
| 8 | Totals | | | |
| 9 | | | | |
| 10 | Meal 2 | | | |
| 11 | Whey Shake ( 1.5 scoops in water | 2 | 30 | 40 |
| 12 | with 2-3 heaped tablespoons of oats) | | | |
| 13 | | | | |
| 14 | | | | |
| 15 | Totals | | | |
| 16 | | | | |
| 17 | Meal 3 | | | |
| 18 | Tandoori Chicken with Rice Dish | | | |
| 19 | | 9 | 45 | 35 |
| 20 | | | | |
| 21 | | | | |
| 22 | Totals | | | |
| 23 | | | | |
| 24 | Meal 4 | | | |
| 25 | Whey Protein Shake with 200ml | | | |
| 26 | water and piece of fruit | 1.5 | 30 | 40 |
| 27 | | | | |
| 28 | | | | |
| 29 | Totals | | | |
| 30 | | | | |
| 31 | Meal 5 | | | |
| 32 | Lean Wholewheat Chapatis with | | | |
| 33 | Beef, chicken or turkey (100-125g | 3.5 | 35 | 30 |
| 34 | cooked weight, in 2-3 chapatis) | | | |
| 35 | | | | |
| 36 | | | | |
| 37 | Totals | | | |
| 38 | | | | |
| 39 | Meal 6 | | | |
| 40 | Whey or Casein Protein Shake | 1.0 | 5 | 40 |
| 41 | 2 scoops in 200ml water | | | |
| 42 | | | | |
| 43 | | | | |
| 44 | Totals | 21 | 175 | 225 |
| 45 | *Daily Total* | 21 | 175 | 205 |
| 46 | *Recommended Totals* | Sat Fat:25g  Un Sat: 25g | 175-225 | 175-220 |

Download Printable Sheets at: **www.bollywood-abs.com**

200

# Low Carb Meal Planner Example

| | A | B | C | D |
|---|---|---|---|---|
| | | | Meals | |
| 1 | **LOW CARB DAY** | **Fats** | **Carbs** | **Protein** |
| 2 | | | | |
| 3 | **Monday** | 20% | 45% | 35% |
| 4 | Egg White Omlette | | | |
| 5 | Tea or Coffee | 5 | 5 | 25 |
| 6 | | | | |
| 7 | | | | |
| 8 | Totals | | | |
| 9 | | | | |
| 10 | Meal 2 | | | |
| 11 | Chicken Chapati | 3.0 | 35 | 30 |
| 12 | (2-3 Chapatis) | | | |
| 13 | | | | |
| 14 | | | | |
| 15 | Totals | | | |
| 16 | | | | |
| 17 | Meal 3 | | | |
| 18 | Pineapple Chicken Kebab | | | |
| 19 | with Rice Dish | 6.5 | 15 | 30 |
| 20 | | | | |
| 21 | | | | |
| 22 | Totals | | | |
| 23 | | | | |
| 24 | Meal 4 | | | |
| 25 | Whey Protein Shake with 200ml | | | |
| 26 | water and piece of fruit | 1.5 | 30 | 40 |
| 27 | | | | |
| 28 | | | | |
| 29 | Totals | | | |
| 30 | | | | |
| 31 | Meal 5 | | | |
| 32 | Tuna Curry with | | | |
| 33 | 2-3 x Wholewheat Chapatis | 4.5 | 40 | 30 |
| 34 | | | | |
| 35 | | | | |
| 36 | | | | |
| 37 | Totals | | | |
| 38 | | | | |
| 39 | Meal 6 | | | |
| 40 | Whey Protein Shake | 1.0 | 5 | 40 |
| 41 | | | | |
| 42 | | | | |
| 43 | | | | |
| 44 | Totals | 21.5 | 130 | 205 |
| 45 | *Daily Total* | 21.5 | 130 | 205 |
| 46 | *Recommended Totals* | Sat Fat:25g  Un Sat: 25g | 125-150 | 175-220 |

Download Printable Sheets at: **www.bollywood-abs.com**

201

# High Carb Vegetarian Example

| | A | B | C | D |
|---|---|---|---|---|
| 1 | **HIGH CARB DAY** | | **Meals** | |
| 2 | | **Fats** | **Carbs** | **Protein** |
| 3 | **Monday** | 20% | 45% | 35% |
| 4,5,6,7 | 80g Wholewheat/Wholegrain Cereal or Oats with 2 scoops of whey, soy or hemp protein in skimmed milk | 4 | 30 | 30 |
| 8 | Totals | | | |
| 9 | | | | |
| 10 | Meal 2 | | | |
| 11,12,13,14 | Maida & Urad Dosa with Tofu, with 1 scoop of whey, soy or hemo in 150ml water | 10 | 40 | 30 |
| 15 | Totals | | | |
| 16 | | | | |
| 17 | Meal 3 | | | |
| 18,19,20,21 | Baked Potato with Spicy Cottage Cheese (add 200g of cottage cheese to this meal) | 5 | 25-30 | 30 |
| 22 | Totals | | | |
| 23 | | | | |
| 24 | Meal 4 | | | |
| 25,26,27,28 | Whey, Soy or Hemp Protein Shake with 200ml water and piece of fruit | 2 | 30 | 40 |
| 29 | Totals | | | |
| 30 | | | | |
| 31 | Meal 5 | | | |
| 32,33,34,35,36 | Vegetable Kashmiri with 2-3 chapatis or rice dish. | 9.5 | 35-40 | 10 |
| 37 | Totals | | | |
| 38 | | | | |
| 39 | Meal 6 | | | |
| 40,41,42,43 | Whey or Casein Protein Shake 2 scoops in 200ml water | 1.0 | 5 | 40 |
| 44 | Totals | 31.5 | 175 | 180 |
| 45 | *Daily Total* | 31.5 | 175 | 180 |
| 46 | *Recommended Totals* | Sat Fat:25g  Un Sat: 25g | 175-225 | 175-220 |

## Download Printable Sheets at: **www.bollywood-abs.com**

# Low Carb Vegetarian Example

| | A | B | C | D |
|---|---|---|---|---|
| | **LOW CARB DAY** | | **Meals** | |
| 1 | | **Fats** | **Carbs** | **Protein** |
| 2 | | | | |
| 3 | **Monday** | 20% | 45% | 35% |
| 4 | Scrambled Tofu Chapati (2 Chapatis) | | | |
| 5 | Tea or Coffee | 22.5 | 30 | 25 |
| 6 | | (18g healthy fat) | | |
| 7 | | | | |
| 8 | Totals | | | |
| 9 | | | | |
| 10 | Meal 2 | | | |
| 11 | Cottage Cheese Snack | 4.5 | 25 | 25 |
| 12 | with Rice Cakes or Brown Idli | | | |
| 13 | | | | |
| 14 | | | | |
| 15 | Totals | | | |
| 16 | | | | |
| 17 | Meal 3 | | | |
| 18 | Stir Fry with Cauliflower and Carrot | | | |
| 19 | 1 scoop of whey, soy or hemp protein | 5 | 14 | 20 |
| 20 | in skimmed milk | | | |
| 21 | | | | |
| 22 | Totals | | | |
| 23 | | | | |
| 24 | Meal 4 | | | |
| 25 | Whey or Soy Protein Shake with 200ml | | | |
| 26 | water and piece of fruit | 3.5 | 30 | 40 |
| 27 | | | | |
| 28 | | | | |
| 29 | Totals | | | |
| 30 | | | | |
| 31 | Meal 5 | | | |
| 32 | Low Fat Aubergine Curry | | | |
| 33 | with 1 scoop of whey or soy protein | 10 | 20 | 25 |
| 34 | in 200ml of skimmed milk | | | |
| 35 | | | | |
| 36 | | | | |
| 37 | Totals | | | |
| 38 | | | | |
| 39 | Meal 6 | | | |
| 40 | Whey or Soy Protein Shake | 1.0 | 5 | 40 |
| 41 | 2 scoops in water | | | |
| 42 | | | | |
| 43 | | | | |
| 44 | Totals | 45.5 | 125 | 170 |
| 45 | *Daily Total* | 45.5 | 125 | 170 |
| 46 | *Recommended Totals* | Sat Fat:25g  Un Sat: 25g | 125-150 | 175-220 |

Download Printable Sheets at: **www.bollywood-abs.com**

# High Carb Western Example

| | A | B | C | D |
|---|---|---|---|---|
| 1 | **HIGH CARB DAY** | | **Meals** | |
| 2 | | **Fats** | **Carbs** | **Protein** |
| 3 | **Monday** | 20% | 45% | 35% |
| 4 | | | | |
| 5 | Meal 1 | | | |
| 6 | Whey Protein Drink (2 scoops) | 4 | 4 | 36 |
| 7 | Shredded Wheat (3 biscuits/non-fat milk) | 1.5 | 45 | 0 |
| 8 | Totals | 5.5 | 49 | 36 |
| 9 | | | | |
| 10 | Meal 2 | | | |
| 11 | Handful of Mixed Nuts | 10 | 0 | 0 |
| 12 | Apple | 1 | 25 | 0 |
| 13 | Coffee non-fat milk, no sugar | 0.2 | 5 | 0 |
| 14 | | | | |
| 15 | Totals | 11.2 | 30 | 0 |
| 16 | | | | |
| 17 | Meal 3 | | | |
| 18 | Baked potato in skin (1 medium) | 0 | 30 | 0 |
| 19 | Steamed mixed veggies (cup) | 0.4 | 10 | 0 |
| 20 | Chicken Breast/s (150g) without skin | 4 | 0 | 40 |
| 21 | | | | |
| 22 | Totals | 4.4 | 40 | 40 |
| 23 | | | | |
| 24 | Meal 4 | | | |
| 25 | Tuna in spring water (150g Drained) | 2 | 0 | 36 |
| 26 | Brown rice (1/2 cup) | 1 | 20 | 0 |
| 27 | Handful of Mixed Nuts | 10 | 0 | 0 |
| 28 | | | | |
| 29 | Totals | 3 | 20 | 36 |
| 30 | | | | |
| 31 | Meal 5 | | | |
| 32 | Whey Protein Drink (2 scoops) | 4 | 4 | 36 |
| 33 | Banana (medium) | 1 | 27 | 0 |
| 34 | non-fat milk (cup) | 0.3 | 9 | 0 |
| 35 | Coffee non-fat milk, no sugar | 0.2 | 5 | 0 |
| 36 | | | | |
| 37 | Totals | 5.5 | 45 | 36 |
| 38 | | | | |
| 39 | Meal 6 | | | |
| 40 | Chicken Breast/s (150g) without skin | 4 | 0 | 40 |
| 41 | Steamed mixed veggies (cup) | 0.4 | 10 | 0 |
| 42 | Baked potato in skin (1 med) | 0 | 30 | 0 |
| 43 | | | | |
| 44 | Totals | 4.4 | 40 | 40 |
| 45 | *Daily Total* | 44 | 224 | 188 |
| 46 | *Recommended Totals* | **40** | **250** | **200** |

Download Printable Sheets at: **www.bollywood-abs.com**

# Low Carb Western Example

| | A | B | C | D |
|---|---|---|---|---|
| 1 | **LOW CARB DAY** | **Meals** | | |
| 2 | | **Fats** | **Carbs** | **Protein** |
| 3 | Tuesday | 25% | 35% | 45% |
| 4 | | | | |
| 5 | Meal 1 | | | |
| 6 | Whey Protein Drink (2 Scoops) | 4 | 4 | 36 |
| 7 | 70g of Oats in water/2% milk | 3 | 45 | 0 |
| 8 | Coffee non-fat milk, no sugar | 0.2 | 6 | |
| 9 | Totals | 7 | 55 | 36 |
| 10 | | | | |
| 11 | Meal 2 | | | |
| 12 | Tuna in spring water (95g) | 1.5 | 0 | 26 |
| 13 | 2 Slices of Wholewheat Bread or Bagel | 1 | 35 | 0 |
| 14 | Glass of Water | | | |
| 15 | | | | |
| 16 | Totals | 2.5 | 35 | 26 |
| 17 | | | | |
| 18 | Meal 3 | | | |
| 19 | Whey Protein Drink (2 scoops) | 4 | 4 | 36 |
| 20 | Handful of mixed nuts or almonds | 10 | 0 | 0 |
| 21 | | | | |
| 22 | | | | |
| 23 | | | | |
| 24 | Totals | 14 | 4 | 36 |
| 25 | | | | |
| 26 | Meal 4 | | | |
| 27 | Tuna in spring water (95g) | 1.5 | 0 | 26 |
| 28 | Wholemeal toast (2 slices) | 3 | 22 | 0 |
| 29 | Coffee non-fat milk, no sugar | 0.2 | 6 | 0 |
| 30 | | | | |
| 31 | Totals | 4.7 | 28 | 26 |
| 32 | | | | |
| 33 | Meal 5 | | | |
| 34 | Whey Protein Drink (1 scoops) | 2 | 2 | 18 |
| 35 | Handful of mixed nuts or almonds | 10 | 0 | 0 |
| 36 | | | | |
| 37 | | | | |
| 38 | Totals | 12 | 2 | 18 |
| 39 | | | | |
| 40 | Meal 6 | | | |
| 41 | Sirloin steak (150g) | 8 | 0 | 35 |
| 42 | Steamed mixed veggies (cup) | 0.4 | 2 | 0 |
| 43 | 100g Sweet Potato | 0 | 20 | 0 |
| 44 | Totals | 8.4 | 22 | 35 |
| 45 | Daily Total | 48.6 | 146 | 177 |
| 46 | Recommended Totals | 50 | 150 | 175 |

Download Printable Sheets at: **www.bollywood-abs.com**

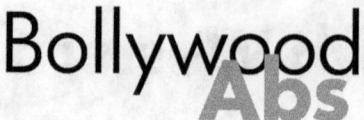

# Bollywood Abs

| CARB DAY | Fats | Carbs | Protein |
|---|---|---|---|
| **DAY:** | | | |
| | | | |
| | | | |
| | | | |
| | | | |
| Totals | | | |
| | | | |
| | | | |
| | | | |
| | | | |
| | | | |
| Totals | | | |
| | | | |
| | | | |
| | | | |
| | | | |
| | | | |
| Totals | | | |
| | | | |
| | | | |
| | | | |
| | | | |
| Totals | | | |
| | | | |
| | | | |
| | | | |
| | | | |
| | | | |
| Totals | | | |
| | | | |
| | | | |
| | | | |
| | | | |
| Totals | | | |
| *Daily Total* | | | |
| *Recommended Totals* | | | |

# **USING** SUPPLEMENTS

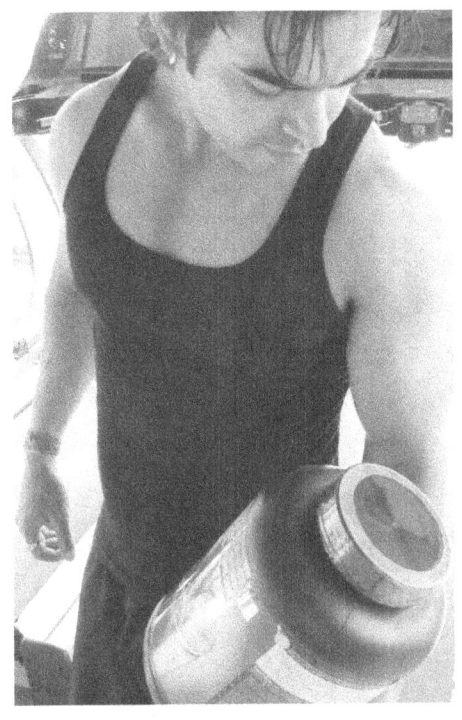

Whilst in India I had the opportunity to speak to many guys with a keen interest in fitness and bodybuilding. What became apparent after speaking to many of them was that there was a genuine reluctance to use supplements, not entirely due to financial reasons, but because of the possible side effects one could encounter. I would like to state that there is no solid evidence to show that whey proteins, creatines, glutamines etc. cause any long terms side effects. These supplements are extremely beneficial to your muscle building efforts and *I strongly encourage there use with this system.*

In fact, any successful nutrition program requires some consumption of quality, scientifically proven supplements. Choosing the right supplements is essential and I will guide you on which ones to use. For optimal results there are five supplements you should consider. For those wishing to add lean muscle, maintain low body fat and define their abdominal muscles a quality **Whey Protein** supplement is essential. As mentioned earlier protein is the building block for muscle and in order to build and maintain muscle you do need an adequate supply throughout the day. Whilst it is important to try and get the majority of your protein from whole foods, whey shakes will make quick and easy meal replacements once or twice daily. Approximately 30-40% of your total protein consumption may come from shakes. Whey Protein is a fast release form of protein meaning that it is absorbed rapidly by the bloodstream, hence it is transported very quickly to your muscles, which is great news for building muscle. Whilst whey protein is ideal during the day, when it comes to night time it's not so beneficial because of its rapid absorption rate. This is where **Casein Protein** comes to the rescue! Casein is a slow release protein which is absorbed at a much slower rate meaning the muscles are fed over the course of a few hours as opposed to minutes with whey protein. Due to this process Casein is perfect to take just before bedtime as it will be released slowly throughout the night.

The second supplement is a **Herbal Fat Burning Supplement**. Although not essential this supplement will certainly increase the fat burning process quite considerably. My advice would be to consider Hydroxycut Hardcore or Hydroxycut Advanced from MuscleTech or Redline from VPX. Thermogenic supplements should be cycled (eg. 4 weeks on, 4 weeks off) so that your body does not become to reliant on them. Some people like to use them for their energy releasing benefits rather than primarily for fat loss. For effective results you should always consume thermogenics on an empty stomach with a glass of water.

The third supplement is **L-Glutamine**. L-Glutamine is a must for anyone looking to maintain muscle size. L-Glutamine acts as a recovery agent for your muscles. Research has proven that when supplemented with, it can help trainees reduce the amount of muscle deterioration that occurs because other tissues that need glutamine will not rob the glutamine stored in the muscle cells. After a high intensity workout, glutamine levels in the body are reduced by as much as 50%. Since the body relies on glutamine as cellular fuel for the immune system, scientific studies suggest that glutamine supplementation can minimize the breakdown of muscle tissue and improve protein metabolism.

For those wishing to add a little weight and extra muscle, **Micronised Creatine** is great supplement. Again creatine is found naturally in many foods and is responsible for providing essential muscle growth. Again our bodies cannot produce sufficient quantities of creatine all day, every day to significantly increase muscle size so supplementation is very beneficial.

The last product is **Green Tea**, this is not so much a supplement, but a natural product, very similar to normal tea. In recent years scientists have studied the benefits of green tea and have made the conclusion that it significantly speeds up the rate at which body fat is burned. Not only is this a great drink, but its very cheap too and comes in a variety of flavors. So, next time you're in the local grocery store be sure to purchase some.

Other supplements to consider are a one-a-day **Multivitamin**. You should know that intense physical stress after exercising causes free radicals to form and can weaken your natural defence system. One a day vitamins help prevent this from happening as they contain a multitude of vitamins and minerals to keep you healthy.

And lastly a **Fish Oil** Supplement. Fish Oil (Healthy Fats) as explained in the book are an easy way to increase your intake of Omega 3 fatty acids.

Besides cholesterol regulation, benefits include anti-inflammatory properties, brain, skin and joint health along with positive effects on body composition and fat loss!

# SUMMARY:

- Don't rely too heavily on supplementation of whey as your main source of protein. Remember to eat lots of fish, poultry and meat.

- Buy a shaker/beaker for easier mixing

- You can make your shakes in the morning, add two ice cubes and they will keep good for a few hours

- You can add honey, blended oats or low fat peanut butter to shakes on training days

- Mix your shakes with either water or skimmed milk

- Don't take fat burning supplements with food. Take only with water on an empty stomach or 1 hour after food. Don't take after 6pm, you'll be awake all night!

- For a good selection of supplements visit: **www.muscleguru.in**

# BURN THE FAT – CARDIO

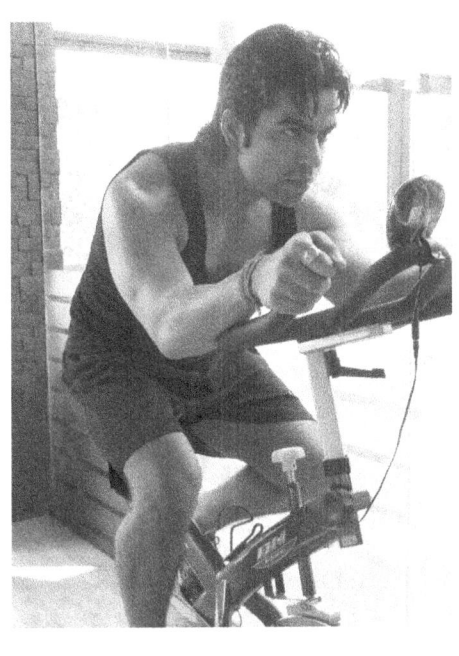

Now I've laid down the fundamentals for your new nutrition plan, now comes the part where it's times to burn those stubborn fat layers. Cardiovascular exercise for some people is a bit of a drag, especially when the results just don't seem to be going the right way. But have you ever thought why you're not seeing results from cardio? More than likely it's because you're consuming more calories than you're burning off! In order to lose fat you have to burn more calories than you consume. All physical activity burns calories, even activities like standing, sitting and even sleeping. The more vigorous an activity, the more calories burned. To lose 1 pound a week, you must burn 3500 *excess* calories, which equates to 500 calories per day over the course of a week.

We have two different types of cardiovascular exercise. Low Intensity and High Intensity. Let's first break these down.

**Low Intensity –** Is an exercise performed at a slower/steady rate. This would most suit a person looking to lose body fat but maintain lean muscle mass. For those of you wanting to keep your hard earned muscle low intensity cardio (60-75% of your Maximum Heart Rate) is most definitely best, since there is greater mobilisation of fat stores and the majority of the calories burned come from fat (no lost muscle).

**High Intensity** – Is an exercise performed at a faster/more intensive rate. This would suit a person whose only concern is to lose body fat and are not too concerned about losing muscle mass in the process. High Intensity Cardio (85-90% of your Maximum Heart Rate) or a 60-75/85-90 split as explained with HIIT in a moment is beneficial because there is less oxidisation of free unbound fatty acids and it burns more calories overall. However, not all the calories come from fat and there may be some muscle mass lost.

**How do I calculate my maximum heart rate (MHR) for Low Intensity and High Intensity cardio?** To calculate your MHR for Low Intensity Cardio first take 220 minus your age. In this instance we will take a 22 year old individual. 220 – 22 = 198 beats per minute. Next, you need to find your target zone (for Low Intensity Cardio this is between 60-75% of your MHR). Multiply your Max Heart Rate (198) by 0.60 and 0.75, which equals 119 – 139 beats per minute. For optimal fat loss you should maintain your heart rate between 119 – 139 beats per minute for the entire duration of the workout. For High Intensity cardio, using the same method simply change the target zone for the High Intensity portion which is 85-90%, so you will take [Your Age], e.g. 22 Year Old = 198 and multiply by 0.85 and 0.90, which equals 169 – 179 beats per minute. You should maintain your heart rate between these two numbers for the duration of the high intensity portion of your workout.

For those choosing a High Intensity Workout, here's a great routine to help burn fat...fast!

**HIIT or High Intensity Interval Training** as its known is just a little different than your typical hour long session on the stationery bike or treadmill. In fact a HIIT session can be fit into a 30 minute session and burn twice the amount of fat than an hour long low intensity session would, and it's been proven. HIIT can be performed with or without cardio machines. It's a form of exercise where you do a short burst and then a high burst of intensity. Not only will a HIIT session speed up your metabolism, but it keeps the metabolic rate increased for hours afterwards. But, you have to push yourself with these workouts or you won't reap the benefits that a HIIT session can offer. Lets take a look at a typical HIIT session and how it works. Lets take for instance a workout on the stationery bike (remember you can use a rower, elliptical, treadmill or go out on a jog or run). You should start off with two minutes of low intensity cycling just to warm those legs up and get that blood circulating. After two minutes have elapsed, its time to crank up the intensity and push hard for a full minute, after that minute has elapsed, it's time to slow things back down again for a minute to catch your breath. After that minute, it's time again to switch things up again to full throttle for another minute. Basically this cycle repeats until 25-30 minutes have elapsed. One minute – low intensity (60-75% of your maximum heart rate) to warm up, then one minute – maximum intensity

(85-90% of your maximum HR), one minute low intensity, one minute maximum intensity and so on. If you're new to cardio, don't even attempt a thirty minute session, you won't even last ten! Just take it easy to begin with, working up to a good twenty-five to thirty minutes after a few weeks. Apply these HIIT sessions to any form of cardio and try to switch things around as much as possible with various equipment. Remember these sessions will be exhaustive and require a great deal of inner strength to make it work effectively.

**Note:** For complete beginners to High Intensity cardio you can make the lower intensity portions longer in duration until you feel confident in reducing them down to one minute.

### When to do cardio

The timing of your cardio sessions is vitally important for maximum results. The best time of all is without doubt first thing in the morning before breakfast (Please Note: It is advisable to consume 10-20g of Whey Protein and 5g of Glutamine 20-30 minutes before cardio to lessen the risk of muscle catabolism (where your body begins to burn muscle) which can happen if cardio is performed with no fuel in the body. Although scientific research has shown that intaking a little protein may mobilize a little less fat, the amount is negligible and the benefits of keeping muscle catabolism at bay does make this practice very important in maintaining muscle.

Not only does a good morning session wake you up, but it sets you up for the rest of the day. Once you make the exercise part of your lifestyle, it will feel more natural to do, than not to, you just have to push yourself that little bit further a make a new exciting step forward to a better body.

Another great time is directly after a weight training session later in the day. When you weight train your glycogen stores become depleted, therefore, when you perform cardio at this time your body burns fat far more effectively. So for best results perform cardio either first thing in the morning or after your weight training session later in the day.

**How much, How Often?**

This very much depends on your activity level during the day. If you have a sedentary job (eg. desk job) then you will need to be looking at a higher amount of cardio compared to someone with an active job (e.g. manual work).

If you just want to maintain your current level of body fat and stay healthy, I recommend 3 - 4 sessions per week. If your goal is maximum fat loss, then I recommend 5-7 sessions per week for some who's activity level during the day would be classed as sedentary. For someone who would consider themselves active during the day, I would recommend 4-5 sessions. Once you reach your desired percentage of body fat, then you could drop down to just 3 - 4 days in order to maintain.

For complete beginners I recommend you work your way up over the course of 12 weeks. Begin with 10 minute sessions 3-4 times weekly. Adding one minute to your sessions each week. Intermediate trainees can begin with 15-17 minute sessions, adding one minute to each session, every week. Advanced trainees can begin with 20-25 minute sessions 5-6 times weekly, increasing to 30 minutes over a period of 6-12 weeks.

HIIT should not be performed for more than 30 minutes in one session. If results remain slow after six weeks you can increase the duration of your sessions or drop your carbs slightly lower. The great thing about HIIT is that you can mix it up, try three minutes fast, one minute slow, 2 minutes fast, 30 seconds slow or even 30 seconds slow, 30 seconds intense. It does take a little experimentation, so try it over the course of a few sessions. You do want to be pleasantly fatigued but not "exhausted" to point of not being able to complete entire session.

I recommend a cool down period of two minutes at the end of your session, a slow jog or walk is fine. In conjunction with the HIIT cardio it is important to keep as active as possible in your everyday life. Walking and other outdoor activities will help considerably in keeping lean, so where possible try to maintain and active lifestyle.

**Low Intensity Workouts**

If you're primary concern is to hold onto hard earned muscle you will need to adopt a low intensity workout (60-75% of your maximum heart rate). Low intensity can be performed on any piece of gym equipment or on a stationery bike or even a walk in your neighborhood. Low intensity is where you perform cardio exercise at a much more manageable pace compared to High Intensity.  One of the most effective workouts is placing a treadmill on a 20-30% gradient and walking for 45-60 minutes in duration.

- Stationery Bike cycling for 45 minutes at 60-75% of your maximum heart rate is also another very effective workout.

- Swimming is a fantastic low intensity workout since it utilises all the major muscle groups of the arms, trunk and legs.

## Which Cardio Exercise Burns the Most Calories?

Below are the top cardio exercises which burn the most calories in 30 minutes. These are great alternatives routines to mix things up a little.

KEY: ||||||||| = HIGH INTENSITY  ||||||| = LOW INTENSITY

**Step Aerobics** – a favorite cardio exercise preferred by women. Step Aerobics mainly target your legs, hips and glutes, and can burn approx. 400 calories in 30 minutes. |||||||||

**Cycling** - stationary or outdoors is a great cardio exercise, depending on resistance and speed can burn 250 to 400 calories in 30 minutes. ||||||||| |||||||

**Swimming** - like cross-country skiing is an excellent cardio exercise as it is a full body workout. Doing the breast stroke can burn approx. 400 calories in 30 minutes. |||||||

**Cross Trainer** - this is an incredible cardio workout as it involves both upper and lower body. A 145 lb person can burn approx 330 calories in 30 minutes. |||||||||

**Running** - Running is an excellent cardio workout because all you need is a pair of quality running shoes. Running burns serious calories. A 145 LB person can easily burn 300 calories in 30 minutes. |||||||||

**Elliptical Trainer** - is a great way to build endurance. A 145 LB person can burn approximately 300 calories in 30 minutes. ||||||| ||||||

**Rowing** - is both a great cardio exercise as well as giving your arms an incredible workout. 145 LB person can burn about 300 calories in 30 minutes. |||||||

**Walking** - Brisk walking is a less strenuous form of cardio exercise. Walking can burn up to 180 calories in 30 minutes. Sprinting, adding hills or an incline can increase amount of calories burned. ||||||

**HIIT Workouts**

1. Jump Rope - This is one of the simplest, yet most effective exercises one can do. In just 15 to 20 minutes, jumping rope will give you an unparalleled total body workout. Jump rope is ideal for cardiovascular endurance and enhances performance in virtually any sport - tennis, basketball, football, skiing, volleyball and more. This simple exercise is also great for eye-hand coordination, lateral movement, foot and hand speed and agility. As many as 500 calories can be burned in a 20 minute period…that's if you can last that long!! |||||||

2. Sprinting - Sprinting not only burns HUGE amounts of calories, it also keeps your metabolism flying for hours after. Sprinting combined with running / jogging can bring amazing results. |||||||

3. Spinning - These high-intensity workouts to music simulate a challenging bike ride, complete with hills, valleys and varying speeds, all dictated by the gym group instructor. |||||||

# Calories Burned from Daily Activities

| Activity | 125 - 174 pounds | 175 - 250 pounds | 250 + pounds |
|---|---|---|---|
| Necessities | Calorie Values for 10 Minutes of Activity | | |
| Sleeping | 10 | 14 | 20 |
| Sitting and Watching Television | 10 | 14 | 18 |
| Sitting and Talking | 15 | 21 | 30 |
| Dressing or Washing | 26 | 37 | 53 |
| Standing | 12 | 16 | 24 |
| Locomotion | Calorie Values for 10 Minutes of Activity | | |
| Walking Downstairs | 56 | 78 | 111 |
| Walking Upstairs | 146 | 202 | 288 |
| Walking at 2 miles per hour | 29 | 40 | 58 |
| Walking at 4 miles per hour | 52 | 72 | 102 |
| Running at 5.5 miles per hour | 90 | 125 | 178 |
| Running at 7 miles per hour | 118 | 164 | 232 |
| Running at 12 miles per hour | 164 | 228 | 326 |
| Cycling at 5.5 miles per hour | 42 | 58 | 83 |
| Cycling at 13 miles per hour | 89 | 124 | 178 |
| Housework | Calorie Values for 10 Minutes of Activity | | |
| Making Beds | 32 | 46 | 65 |
| Washing Floors | 38 | 53 | 75 |
| Washing Windows | 35 | 48 | 69 |
| Dusting | 22 | 31 | 44 |
| Preparing a Meal | 32 | 46 | 6 |
| Light Gardening | 30 | 42 | 59 |
| Weeding Garden | 49 | 68 | 98 |

| Activity | 125 - 174 pounds | 175 - 250 pounds | 250 + pounds |
|---|---|---|---|
| Sedentary Occupations | Calorie Values for 10 Minutes of Activity | | |
| Sitting Writing | 15 | 21 | 30 |
| Light Office Work | 25 | 34 | 50 |
| Standing with Light Activity | 20 | 28 | 40 |
| Typing with Computer | 19 | 27 | 39 |
| Light Physical Labor Occupations | Calorie Values for 10 Minutes of Activity | | |
| Assembly Line | 20 | 28 | 40 |
| Auto Repair | 35 | 48 | 69 |
| Carpentry | 32 | 44 | 64 |
| Bricklaying | 28 | 40 | 57 |
| Farming Chores | 32 | 44 | 64 |
| House Painting | 29 | 40 | 58 |
| Heavy Physical Labor Occupations | Calorie Values for 10 Minutes of Activity | | |
| Pick and Shovel Work | 56 | 78 | 110 |
| Chopping Wood | 60 | 84 | 121 |
| Dragging Logs | 158 | 220 | 315 |
| Sports | Calorie Values for 10 Minutes of Activity | | |
| Baseball | 39 | 54 | 78 |
| Basketball | 58 | 82 | 117 |
| Bowling (non-stop) | 56 | 78 | 111 |
| Canoeing at 4 miles per hour | 90 | 128 | 182 |
| Dancing (moderate) | 35 | 48 | 69 |
| Dancing (vigorous) | 48 | 66 | 94 |
| Football | 69 | 96 | 137 |
| Golfing | 33 | 48 | 68 |
| Horseback Riding | 56 | 78 | 112 |
| Ping-Pong | 32 | 45 | 64 |
| Racquet ball | 75 | 104 | 144 |
| Swimming (Backstroke) | 32 | 45 | 64 |
| Swimming (Crawl) | 40 | 56 | 80 |
| Tennis | 56 | 80 | 115 |
| Volleyball | 43 | 65 | 94 |

# NOW IT'S YOUR TURN...

So there it is, the key principles of my Bollywood Abs System. Each element I've mentioned is a piece that makes up the jigsaw puzzle I spoke about at the beginning of the book. If you leave one piece out, the puzzle will not be complete. It's the same for the program. You should by 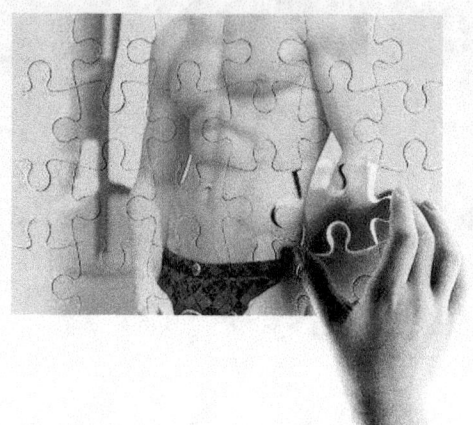 now be ready to make some important new changes in your life. Now you can see how each piece of the jigsaw is put together, it's your turn. By reading all the information provided in the book you now need to apply all the training, nutrition and exercise principles and get to work!. Make notes, fill in a journal to track your progress, write down this weeks shopping list, print off the training sheets and get ready to begin your plan.

Be sure you have carefully read all the information and ensure all your questions are answered. Set yourself targets for the coming week, what days you'll train, what times you'll eat and how long you'll rest. Ensure you have some basic equipment to begin your plan (either a gym membership or a basic bench with dumbbells or a barbell) Cardio wise, you can either use a stationery bike, treadmill, skipping rope, rower or elliptical machine, or go for a run or walk!

Just as important is to have some form of back up plan, just in case work or social commitments cause an unscheduled side track from the program. Ensure you always have water and some form of protein snack to hand just in case something may arise. Careful planning and preparation are crucial aspects of any training program and will not only help keep track of your progress, but will give you the ability to carefully scrutinize aspects which may or may not be working. Remember to keep positive throughout, a positive mental attitude will bring out your very best.

Dedication, commitment and sheer determination will create abs and a body you never thought possible. As I mentioned in the introduction, great bodies are not just reserved for move stars, celebrities, athletes, models or sports stars, we all have the ability to completely change our physique. It's now time for you to apply the program, apply the diet and apply the exercise, in return a great new body is in the making.

The road ahead is going to have ups and downs, but trust me when I say 'You can do it!'. Never give in and never give up. I know many, many Indian guys who use the principles and diet I have provided in this book and they have created great bodies. But please remember this... Diet, Diet, Diet!  If you do not use my healthier approach to your diet you will not succeed. You MUST make a commitment to change and adopt the meals I have designed in this book, it will ultimately lead to your success or failure!

I hope this book will help you realise your dreams and take your body to the next level. As I sit and write this final chapter of the book I have chosen to do so at one of the most magnificent places I have ever been too – The Taj Mahal. Where better to gather my final thoughts on writing the book and reminisce of my time here in India. An experience that will last a lifetime, For now all that is left for me to say is Goodbye and Good Luck! And remember........."abs are made in the kitchen....not in the gym!"

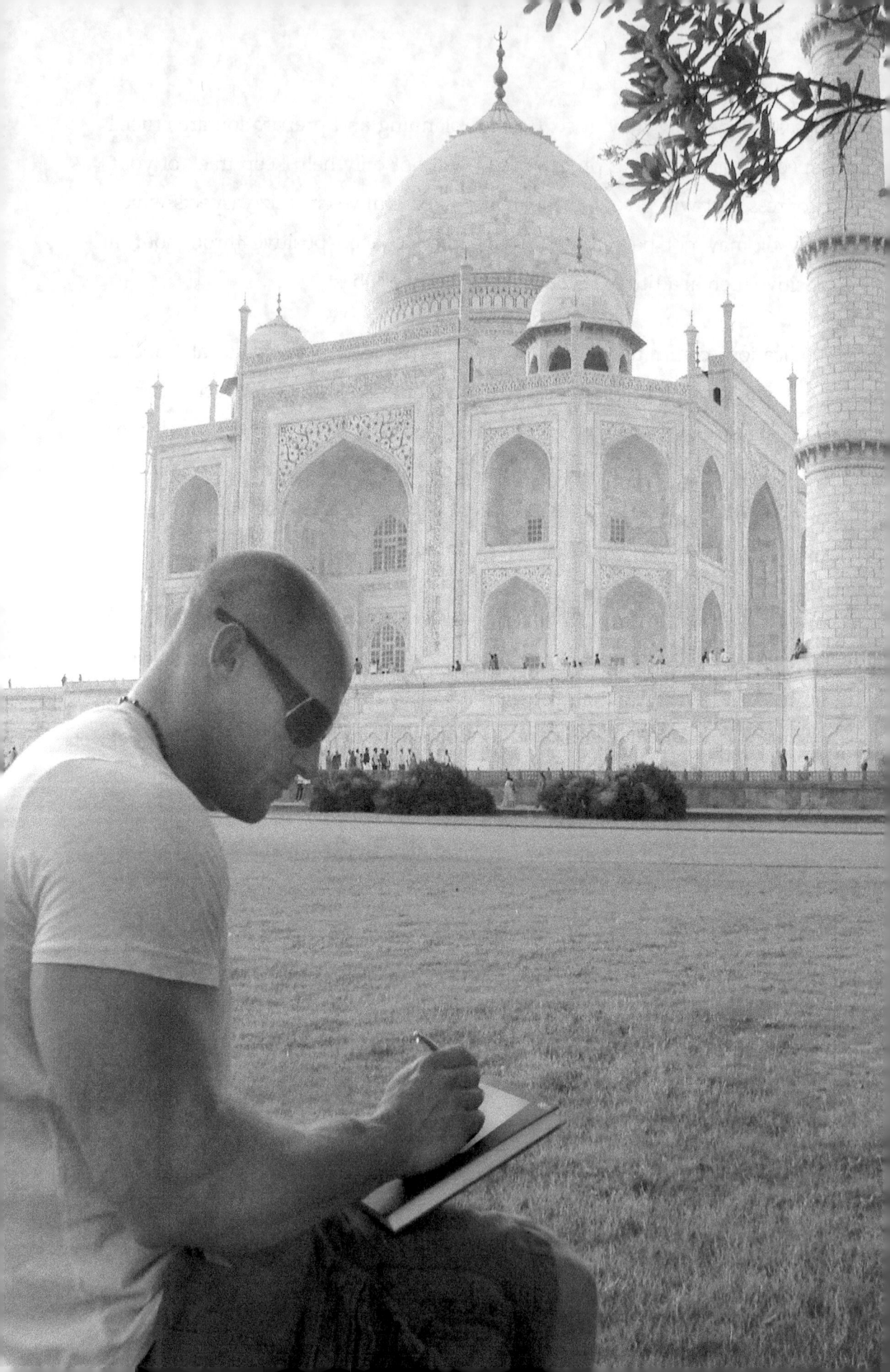

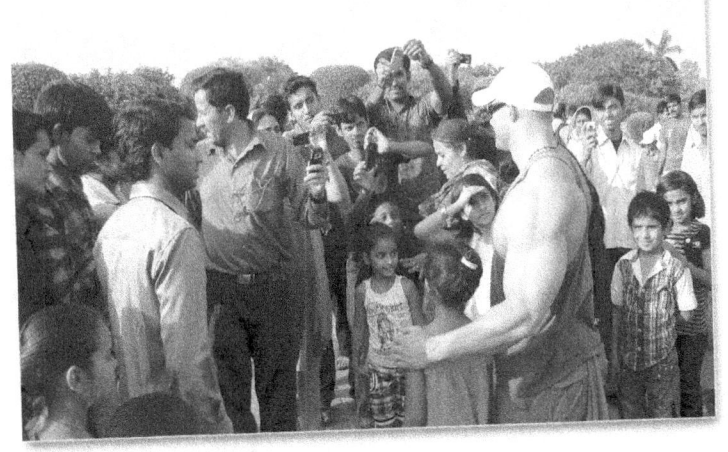

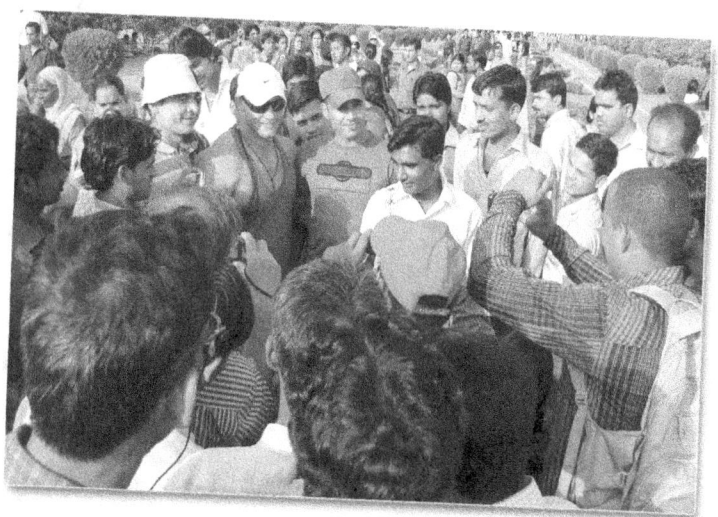

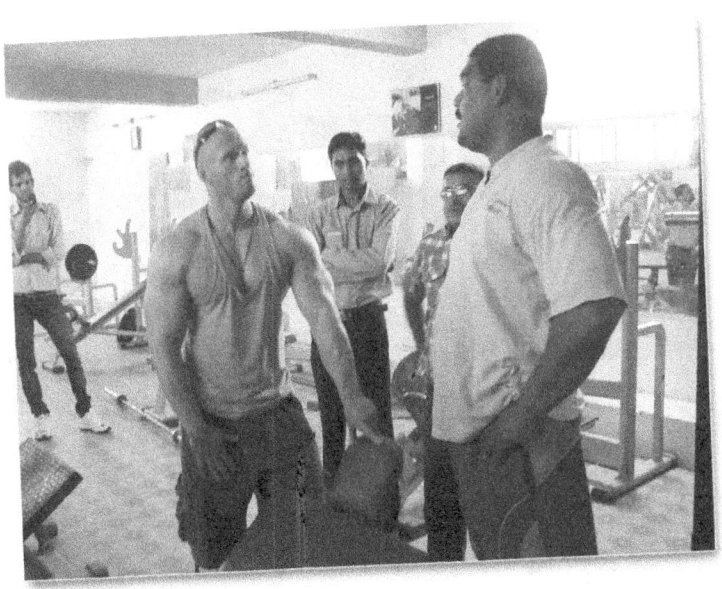

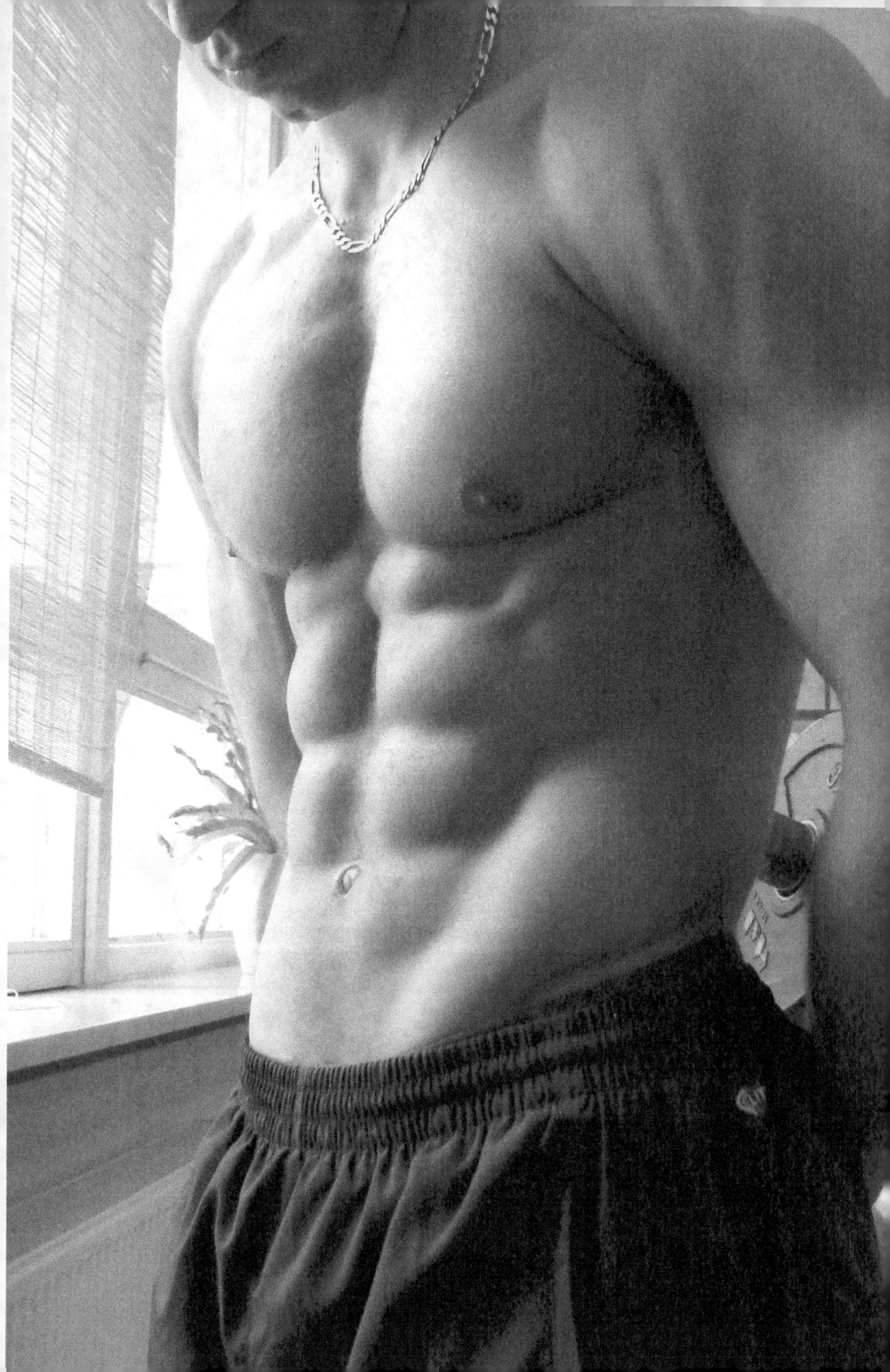

# BOLLYWOOD ABS WORKOUT

The Bollywood Abs workout will focus on the three different sections of the abdominals - the uppers, lowers and side obliques. Before moving onto the exercises let me first explain a little about the abdominals.

As I mentioned in the introduction, far too many people buy into these ab training gadgets and contraptions with hopes of achieving rock hard abs in 14 days! I'd be surprised if anyone had actually achieved a six pack from using them alone. Most people don't even know what the ab muscles are, how they function and how they should be trained in order for them to be visible. One common pitfall with so many trainees is that they think they only need to work one area of the abdominals in order to achieve a nice set of abs! Crunches alone won't cut it. You need to **hit your abs from every angle** to carve out those cuts and grooves. Let's take a look at the different sections of the abdominal wall in a little more detail.

## THE UPPER ABS

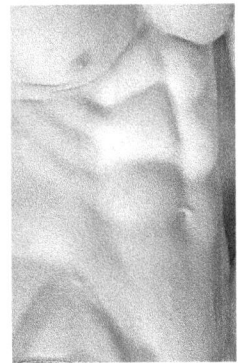

The upper area of the Rectus Abdominis is a large muscle that extends across your stomach from the rib cage down to your hips. The six prominent muscles in the stomach 'six pack' are the result of strong bands of connective tissue that cut into the rectus abdominis muscle. The more developed this muscle becomes, the more deeper the grooves and cut appearance you will see. Abs do come in various shapes and sizes. Not all abs are perfectly formed and the appearance and look of individual ab muscles comes down to genetics, but one thing is certain, we all have six abdominal muscles under that layer of fat and for the very fortunate, eight! Yes, some people have eight abs (eight-pack). The most effective exercises for this area are all types of crunches and exercises where the shoulders are lifted off the floor. When the upper abs are worked hard you will feel a burning sensation, this means you've exercised your abs to maximum intensity.

## THE LOWER ABS

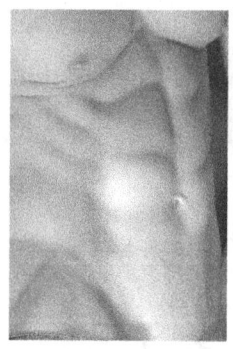 Whilst the lower abs are a continuation of the rectus abdominis found in the upper abs both regions do require isolation from different exercises. Focusing on the lower region will bring out the much sought after v-cut in the abs and produce the lower two abdominal muscles to complete the 'six pack' look. The lower ab area is activated during exercises that primarily involve lifting the legs off the floor. When performing lower ab workouts it is during this time that many people feel lower back discomfort. This is due to the hip flexor muscles taking much of the strain. This can be avoided by not over-working your lower abs. Because the lower abs fatigue much more quickly than the uppers it is important not to try and force reps out once you've reached failure, it is at this point that the hip flexors will take over and cause the back pain.

## THE OBLIQUES

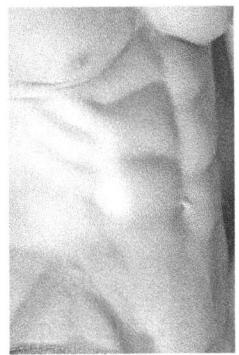 The obliques are your side abdominals and are often an area that is neglected. Having a well defined set of obliques when combined with a firm six pack really does complete the picture. Exercises that target the obliques include those that twist and also focus on being trained separately, most notably oblique crunches. It is important not to over-train the obliques as this could cause your waist to thicken up, giving the appearance of a wider stomach! Something you don't want.

Ok, now it's time to select some exercises to make up your ab workouts. You should pick one section for each workout, for example, ONLY Upper Abs will be exercised on a Monday, ONLY Lower Abs on a Wednesday and ONLY Side Obliques on a Friday. That's three separate Ab Workouts per week. We have three different levels which you should follow. Beginner, Intermediate and Advanced. Here is how you should approach the levels:

If you are completely new to Abdominal Exercise you should begin with the Beginners exercises for 2-5 weeks and then progress to the Intermediate exercises on week 5 or 6, depending on how comfortable you feel with them. Again, it should be remembered that more or harder exercising will not make your abs more prominent, diet is the key.

If you are familiar with abdominal exercise and currently incorporate exercises into your workouts, you may select any of the beginner or intermediate exercises and progress to the Advanced level exercises after

3 weeks. If you have very low body fat levels and are familiar with abdominal exercise you may incorporate our Advanced exercises in conjunction with any from the beginner or intermediate level.

## REPS & SETS

If you're a complete beginner to abdominal exercise you should perform three different exercises (3 sets each), for a total of 9 sets. You will perform 1 set of each of the 3 exercises and then repeat the routine a further two times. Reps should be kept in the range of 10-15 for each exercise.

## AFTER THREE WEEKS OR FOR INTERMEDIATE TRAINEES

## GOING TO FAILURE

After three weeks of ab exercising you can begin to take your repetitions to 'failure' or 'fatigue'. This means you do not set yourself rep ranges. Failure will be reached when your abs start to 'burn'. This will ensure you're taking your exercises to maximum intensity. Some exercises will be hard to take to failure, so where possible incorporate weighted or resistance based exercises to bring down rep ranges. If you find you can perform more than 30-40 repetitions easily of any given exercise, add resistance. A good idea would be to incorporate one exercise where you can easily reach failure, another exercise which you can perform a good 20 repetitions and another exercise where you can use weight or resistance.

Correct execution of the exercises is paramount. Ensure you read the information on each exercise very carefully and copy the exact placement shown in the photos. To avoid back strain or injury ensure your back remains flat throughout exercises.

Place emphasis on your abdominals throughout the movements. Keeping the abs tight will ensure you are placing pressure on them.

**PLEASE REMEMBER**

For best results you should cycle exercises every 3-4 weeks to provide new stimulation for your abs.

**IMPORTANT**

If you have a sizeable amount of body fat covering your abdominals, I would suggest concentrating more on cardio exercise to aid fat reduction. Ab workouts may still be incorporated, but should be used to strengthen and prime your abs for more rigorous workouts that will be incorporated when you see a more prominent reduction in body fat.

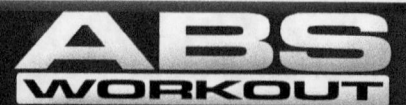

## WEEK 1-4 - BEGINNER    MONDAY

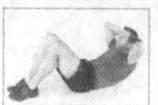
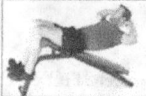
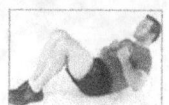

**CRUNCH**     **DECLINE CRUNCH**     **WEIGHTED CRUNCHES**

OR       OR       OR

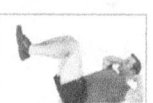
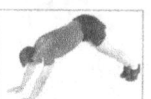
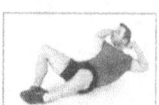

**TUCK CRUNCH**     **BUTT RAISES**     **BUTTERFLY CRUNCH**

### UPPER ABS ONLY

- Perform exercise 1, once, the move onto exercise 2 and perform once, then move onto exercise 3 and perform once. You will repeat this routine 3 times (Total 9 sets)

- Maintain strict form throughout

- Complete beginners should aim for 10-15 reps

- After two weeks you should aim to 'FAILURE'

- If you find weighted crunches too difficult just place your hands on your chest.

- FEEL your abs work on every repetition

## WEEK 1-4 - BEGINNER    WEDS

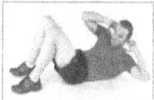
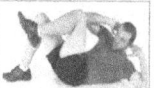
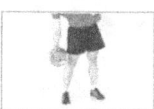

**OBLIQUE CRUNCH**     **CROSS CRUNCH**     **SIDE BENDS**

OR       OR       OR

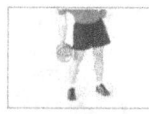
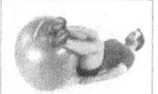
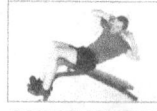

**SIDE BENDS**     **HIP ROLLS**     **DECLINE OBLIQUE**

### OBLIQUE ABS ONLY

- Perform exercise 1, once, the move onto exercise 2 and perform once, then move onto exercise 3 and perform once. You will repeat this routine 3 times (Total 9 sets)

- Maintain strict form throughout

- Complete beginners should aim for 10-15 reps

- After two weeks you should aim to 'FAILURE'

- Use a light weight on the side bends

- FEEL your abs work on every repetition

## WEEK 1-4 - BEGINNER    FRIDAY

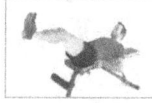
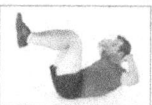
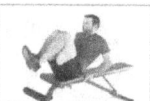

**LEG RAISES**     **DOUBLE CRUNCH**     **PULL-INS**

OR       OR       OR

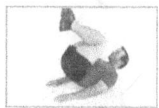
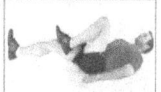
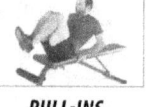
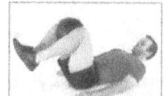

**REVERSE CRUNCH**     **LEG PUSHAWAY**     **MED BALL REV. CURLS**

### LOWER ABS ONLY

- Perform exercise 1, once, the move onto exercise 2 and perform once, then move onto exercise 3 and perform once. You will repeat this routine 3 times (Total 9 sets)

- Maintain strict form throughout

- Complete beginners should aim for 10-15 reps

- After two weeks you should aim to 'FAILURE'

- FEEL your abs work on every repetition

# INTERMEDIATE **WORKOUT**

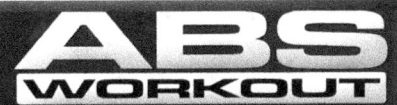

## WEEK 5-8 - INTERMEDIATE — MONDAY

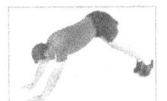
**BUTT RAISES**

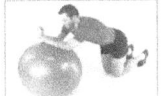
**BALL/BARBELL ROLL-OUT**

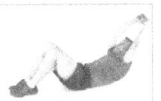
**CRUNCH  EX. ARMS**

*OR*       *OR*       *OR*

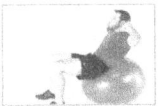
**BALL CRUNCH**

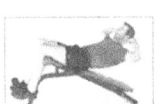
**WEIGHTED CRUNCH**

**DECLINE CRUNCH**

### UPPER ABS ONLY

- Perform exercise 1, once, the move onto exercise 2 and perform once, then move onto exercise 3 and perform once. You will repeat this routine 3 times (Total 9 sets)

- Maintain strict form throughout

- You should aim for FAILURE on all exercises, this is where your abs will burn.

- Feel free to mix up your workouts with other exercises.

- FEEL your abs work on every repetition

## WEEK 5-8 - INTERMEDIATE — WEDS

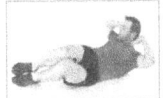
**OB. CRUNCH LEGS BENT**

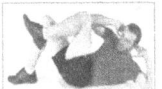
**CROSS CRUNCH**

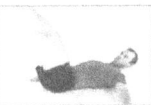
**PENDULUM**

*OR*       *OR*       *OR*

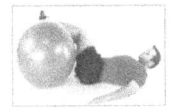
**HIP ROLLS ON BALL**

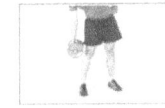
**SIDE BENDS**

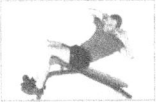
**DECLINE OBLIQUE**

### OBLIQUE ABS ONLY

- Perform exercise 1, once, the move onto exercise 2 and perform once, then move onto exercise 3 and perform once. You will repeat this routine 3 times (Total 9 sets)

- Maintain strict form throughout

- Complete beginners should aim for 10-15 reps

- After two weeks you should aim to 'FAILURE'

- Use a light weight on the side bends

- FEEL your abs work on every repetition

## WEEK 5-8 - INTERMEDIATE — FRIDAY

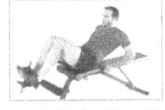
**WEIGHTED PULL-INS**

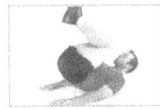
**REVERSE CRUNCH**

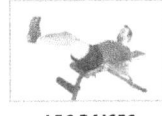
**LEG RAISES**

*OR*       *OR*       *OR*

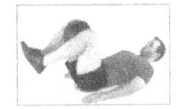
**MED BALL REV. CURLS**

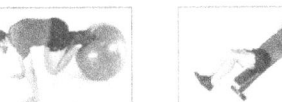
**SWISS BALL PULL-IN**

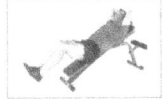
**REVERSE ON DECLINE**

### LOWER ABS ONLY

- Perform exercise 1, once, the move onto exercise 2 and perform once, then move onto exercise 3 and perform once. You will repeat this routine 3 times (Total 9 sets)

- Maintain strict form throughout

- Complete beginners should aim for 10-15 reps

- After two weeks you should aim to 'FAILURE'

- FEEL your abs work on every repetition

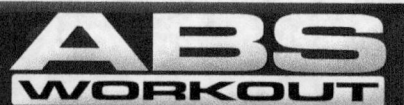

## WEEK 9-12 - ADVANCED · MONDAY

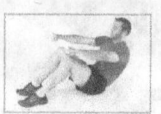
**JANDA SIT UP**

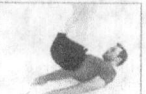
**HIP THRUSTS**

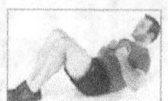
**WEIGHTED CRUNCH**

*OR* · *OR* · *OR*

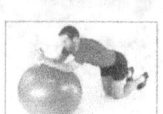
**BALL/BARBELL ROLL-OUT**

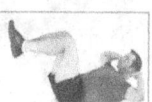
**TUCK CRUNCH**

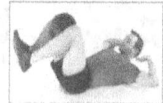
**CLAMSHELL**

### UPPER ABS ONLY

- Perform exercise 1, once, the move onto exercise 2 and perform once, then move onto exercise 3 and perform once. You will repeat this routine 3 times (Total 9 sets)
- Maintain strict form throughout
- You should aim for FAILURE on all exercises, this is where your abs will burn.
- Feel free to mix up your workouts with other exercises.
- FEEL your abs work on every repetition

## WEEK 9-12 - ADVANCED · WEDS

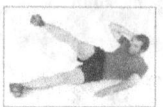
**SIDE JACKNIFE**

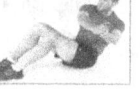
**RUSSSIAN TWIST**

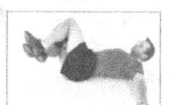
**PENDULUM WITH BALL**

*OR* · *OR* · *OR*

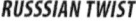
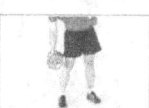
**OB. CRUNCH LEGS BENT**

**SIDE BENDS**

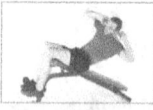
**DECLINE OBLIQUE**

### OBLIQUE ABS ONLY

- Perform exercise 1, once, the move onto exercise 2 and perform once, then move onto exercise 3 and perform once. You will repeat this routine 3 times (Total 9 sets)
- Maintain strict form throughout
- Complete beginners should aim for 10-15 reps
- After two weeks you should aim to 'FAILURE'
- Use a light weight on the side bends
- FEEL your abs work on every repetition

## WEEK 9-12 - ADVANCED · FRIDAY

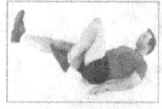
**CYCLE CRUNCH**

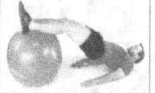
**BENT KNEE BRIDGE**

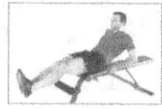
**PULL-INS ON BENCH OR WEIGHTED**

*OR* · *OR* · *OR*

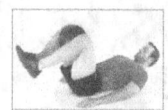
**MED BALL REV. CURLS**

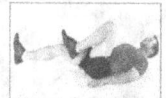
**LEG PUSHAWAY**

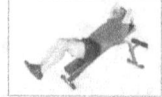
**REVERSE ON DECLINE**

### LOWER ABS ONLY

- Perform exercise 1, once, the move onto exercise 2 and perform once, then move onto exercise 3 and perform once. You will repeat this routine 3 times (Total 9 sets)
- Maintain strict form throughout
- Complete beginners should aim for 10-15 reps
- After two weeks you should aim to 'FAILURE'
- FEEL your abs work on every repetition

# UPPER ABS

### Crunch

Lie flat on your back with your feet flat on the ground. Place your hands lightly on either side of your head keeping your elbows out. Push your back to the floor to isolate your abdominal muscles. Begin to roll your shoulders off the floor, keeping your lower back firmly on the floor. Your 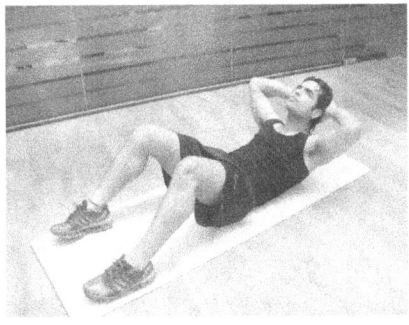 shoulders should come up off the floor about four inches. As always, make sure you let your abs do the work in a slow and controlled manner. As your shoulders come up squeeze those abs in a crunching motion.

### Decline Crunch   Neil's Favorite

Using a decline bench (equipment may vary), position yourself with your feet locked in at the top. Place your hands on either side of your head, without locking your fingers. Raise your body slowly while you contract your abs. Crunch up, bringing your elbows to either side of 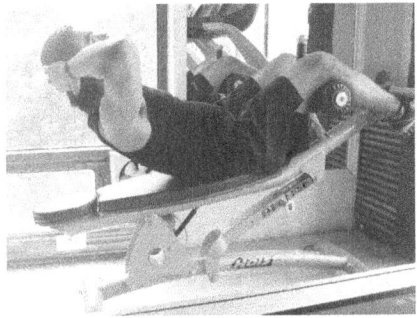 your thighs. At the top of the movement, flex your abs for a one-count and then slowly lower your body back to the starting position. Be sure to keep at least an inch or two of space between your back and the bench at the bottom of the movement.

### Weighted Crunch

Lie flat on the ground with your knees bent and both feet flat on the floor. Place a weight plate flat on your chest, folding your arms across or holding it at each side to hold it in place. Slowly curl your torso forward, raising your head and shoulder blades off the floor and bring 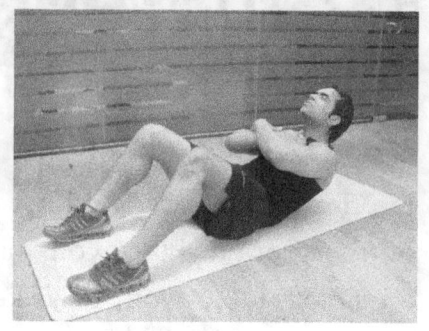 you pelvis towards your head at the same time. Pause for two seconds, then slowly lower yourself back to the floor, resisting the weight on the way down.

### Tuck Crunch

Lie on the floor with your hands either crossed over your chest or behind your head. Bend your knees and hips to form right angles. Keep your lower legs parallel to the floor and your feet crossed. Lift your shoulder blades a few inches off the floor by curling up. Slowly 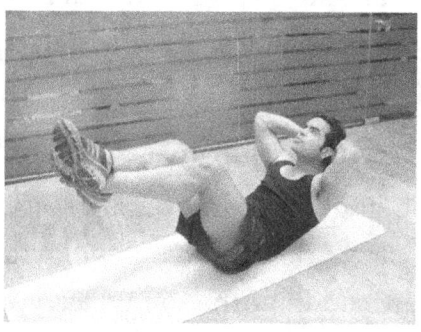 return to the starting position after squeezing your abs.

### Butterfly Crunch

Lie on your back with the soles of your feet together, as close to your body as possible, and your knees bent out to the sides. Place your hands behind your head or crossed over your chest. Keeping your back flat on floor and your stomach muscles contracted, exhale and curl your 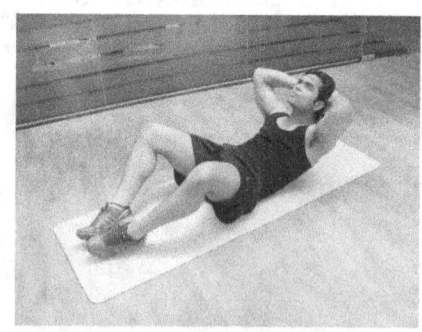 chest up a few inches off the floor toward your legs.

## Butt Raises

Start in a push up-like position with your elbows and forearms flat on the ground and your legs stretched out straight, keeping your knees off the ground. Lift your butt upward, putting the emphasis on your abs to do the lifting.

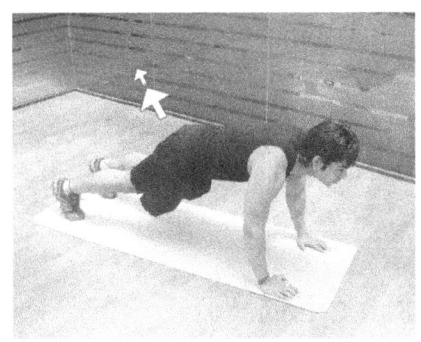

## Ab Rollouts

Select a light barbell and place on the ground. Standing above the barbell, bend down keeping your legs straight and grab the barbell with both hands (shoulder width apart). Next, slowly roll your torso forward while keeping your arms fully extended in a straight and locked

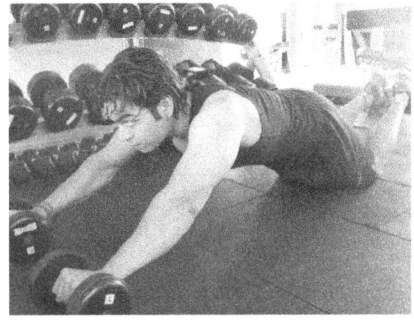

position. Allow yourself to roll forward until your torso becomes parallel to the floor. Be sure that your arms stay perpendicular to the floor so as not to cause unnecessary stress on your shoulders and elbows. When returning to the start position, the emphasis should be on raising your rear end as high as possible back into the straight legged starting position.

## Cable Crunch   Neil's Favorite

Sit on your heels. The resistance from the cable must be above you and over your head—use a rope attachment or handles for your grip. Kneel down, facing away from the resistance with your hands at the sides of your head and your elbows tucked close to your body.

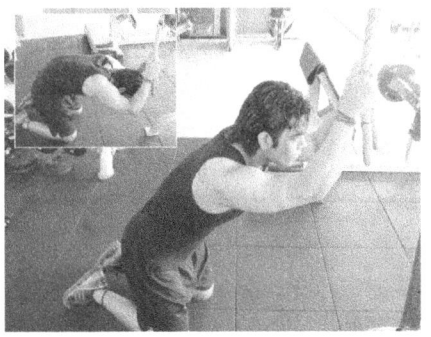

Keeping your arms stationary, use your ab muscles to pull your chest towards the floor. Curl your spine forward and down as you pull in your abs. Once you've curled your body as far as it will go, hold for 1 second and then slowly return to the starting position.

**Ball Crunch**

Sit on top of an exercise ball, feet placed firmly on the floor. Slide forward, rolling the bottom half of your glutes off the ball, until your lower back is centered atop of the ball. Place your hands at the sides of your head. Crunch your upper body forward, rolling your shoulders toward 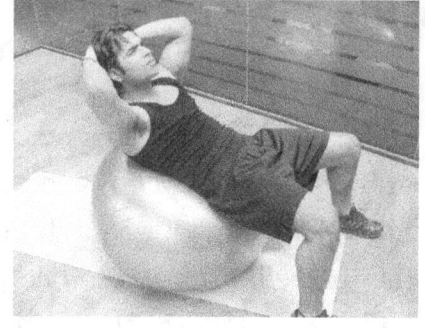 your hips. Squeeze your abs at the top of the movement, lower and repeat.

**Janda Sit Up**

It is beneficial to use a partner for this exercise. Lie on the floor with your knees bent to 90 degrees and your feet flat. Your partner will hold on to your legs about halfway between your ankles and knees and apply steady pressure as if trying to pull your feet off the floor. 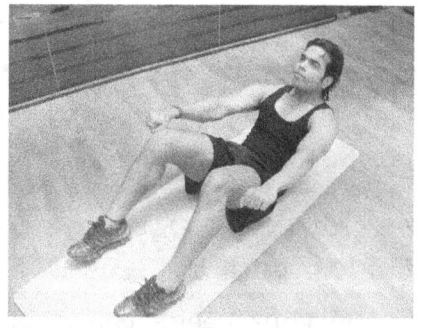 Don't let him. Tighten your glutes and hamstrings to keep your soles flat on the floor. Keep your arms at your sides and slowly sit up without jerking. Squeezing the hamstrings and glutes takes the hip flexors out of the movement.

## Hip Thrusts

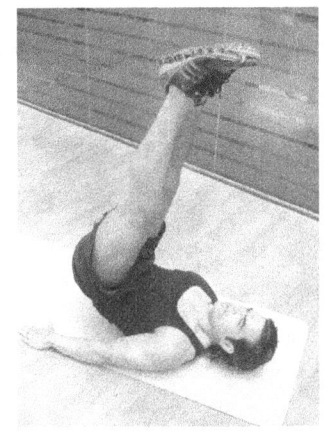

Lie face up on the floor with your hips bent 90 degrees, legs straight up in the air and perpendicular to the floor. Gently press your lower back into the floor while keeping your torso tight. Keep your arms out wide and flat on the floor for balance, palms down. Lightly press your hands "into" the floor to assist in balancing your body during the movement. Inhale deeply and hold your breath as you lift your hips and legs straight up toward the ceiling. When you reach the top (the range of motion should be only a few inches), hold for a brief second, then exhale as you slowly lower your hips/legs.

## Clamshell

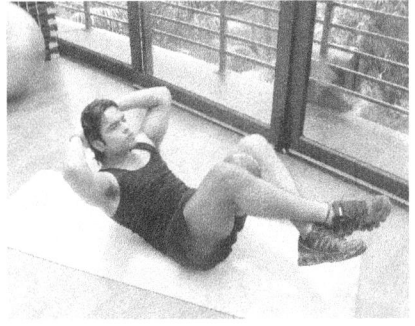

Sit on a mat and place a stability ball between your legs (at your knees or ankles). Squeezing the ball in place, lie back onto the floor, keeping your feet just off the ground, knees bent. Make sure your lower back stays planted and your abs are tight. Place your hands lightly behind your ears in a crunch position. Exhale as you simultaneously lift your shoulders off the ground and your knees into your chest to perform a double crunch. Then inhale as you slowly return to start to complete one rep. Don't let momentum swing your knees up for you. Be sure your hands are not lifting your upper body-- concentrate on using abs.

# OBLIQUE EXERCISES

### Oblique Crunch

Lie on your back with your hands behind your head so that your fingers rest behind your ears. Open your elbows up and out to the side. Keep your shoulder blades on the floor. Lift your knees up and together as you bring them to one side. Keep them stacked on top of each 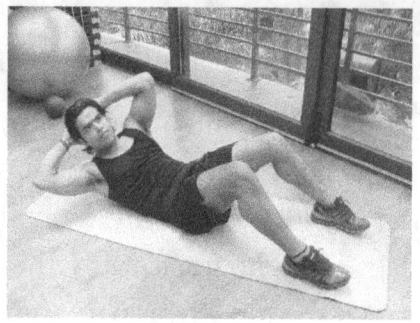 other. Using slow and controlled movements, raise your upper torso directly off the floor. Continue to pull the left shoulder up and toward the right knee until the abdominal muscles are fully contracted. Slowly return to the start position and repeat. Be sure to keep your chin up as if you are holding an orange. This will help to prevent neck injury. Alternate to the other side after completion of the left obliques.

### Cross Crunch

Lie on your back and bend your knees about 60 degrees and keep your feet flat on the floor. Place your hands loosely behind your head. Curl up and bring your right elbow and shoulder across your body while bring your left knee in toward your left shoulder at the same 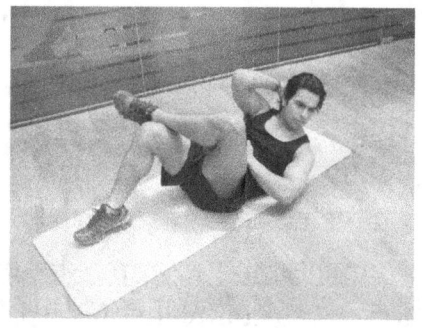 time. Reach with your elbow and try to touch your knee. Do one side for all your reps, then switch to the other side.

## Side Bends

Stand straight with one arm behind your head and the other holding a light dumbbell. Bend sideways holding your pelvis very firm. First one shoulder should bend down toward the floor. When you reach a point where you cannot bend further, inhale, hold your breath and raise yourself back to the erect starting position exhaling when you reach the vertical position. Repeat this movement for X reps before switching to the opposite shoulder.

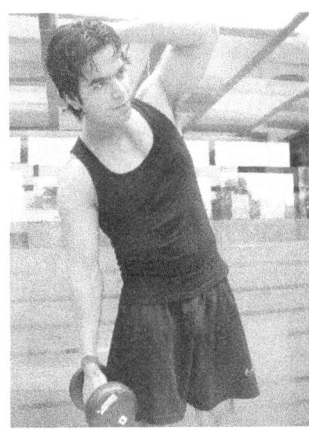

## Pendulum

Lying on the floor, have your legs extended straight up. Arms should be straight out to the sides, head resting on the floor. Exhale and motion with your legs towards your left side. When you reach a couple feet off the floor, inhale, and bring legs back up to center.

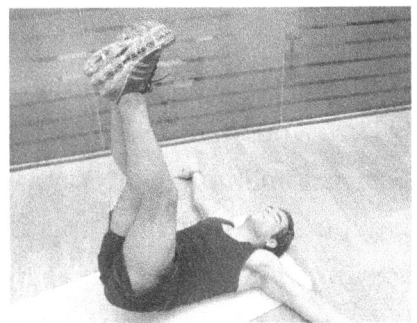

Continue with the same motion on the right side. This should be one continual motion without any pauses. Return to center for one complete rep.

## Hip Rolls on Ball

Simply lie on the floor with your feet firmly positioned atop the swiss ball. Your knees should be bent at a 90 degree angle. Place your hands on the ground. Once you are comfortable with your position, rotate your hips to your right, you'll feel the ball move slightly. As you

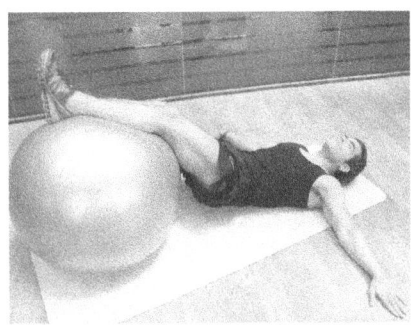

roll your hips be sure to squeeze those abs and obliques in the process.

Return to the start position and repeat. After one set, perform in the opposite direction.

### Side Jack-Knife

Lying on your right side and keeping your left leg over your right one, place your right hand in a comfortable spot and clasp your left hand behind your head. Bring your torso and left leg toward each other as you pull with your obliques. Squeeze for a moment and 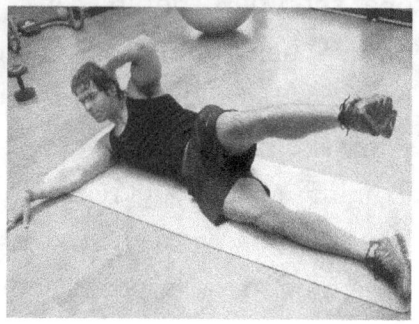 return to the starting position. You can use ankle weights to make it tougher!

### Russian Twist

Secure your feet either by placing them under something that won't move or by having a partner hold them. Start in the position shown above, leaning slightly back and clasping your hands in front of you. Moving only at the trunk, rotate to one side. At the end of your range of 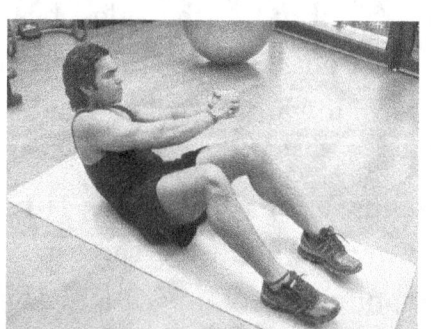 motion, quickly reverse the movement and rotate to the opposite side. Repeat in a rapid fashion for the full number of reps. You can also hold a weight or medicine ball to increase the difficulty.

# **LOWER** AB EXERCISES

### Leg Raises

Lie flat on your back on a bench with your legs off the end. Place your hands back next to your head and grab the edge of the bench. Keeping your legs as straight as possible, raise your legs as high as possible, making sure that your abs are doing the work. Lower legs back down to the start position and repeat.

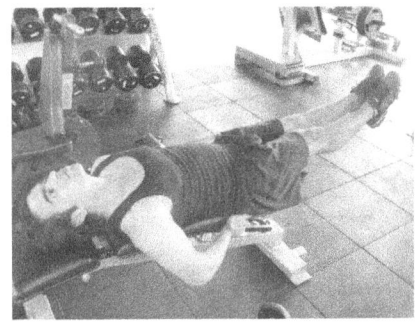

### Double Crunch

Lie as shown. Head should be in a neutral position with a space between chin and chest. Hands behind head and knees bent at 90 degrees. Leading with the chin and chest towards the ceiling, contract the abdominals and raise shoulders off floor or bench. During the crunch, also bring knees towards chest.

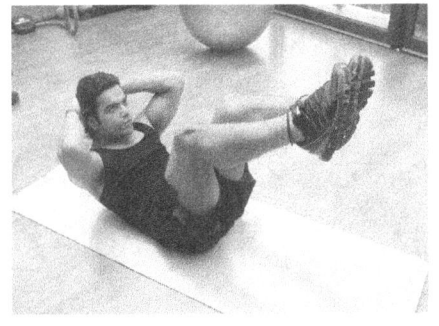

### Reverse Crunch

Lie on the floor on a mat on your back. Place your arms by your sides with your feet up and your thighs perpendicular to the floor. Using your lower abs, bring your knees to your chest while simultaneously tucking your chin to your chest. Return slowly to the starting position and repeat.

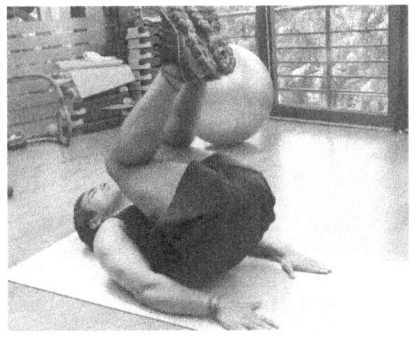

## Pull-Ins

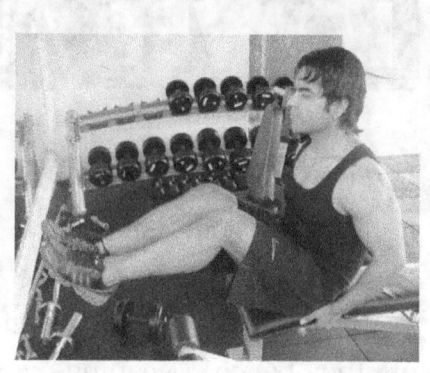

Sit on a flat bench with your legs off the end. Place your hands to your sides, grasping the edge of the bench with each hand. Extend your legs straight out and lean your back at a 45 degree angle. Bring your knees in toward your midsection, making sure that your abs are doing the work in a slow and controlled fashion. Return to the starting position.

## Weighted Pull-Ins

As above, this is a variation of the Pull-In but using a weight to place more demand on the abs. Sit on a flat bench with your legs off the end and a dumbbell positioned in-between your feet. Place your hands to your sides, grasping the edge of the bench with each hand. Extend your legs straight out and lean your back at a 45 degree angle. Bring your knees in toward your midsection, making sure that your abs are doing the work in a slow and controlled fashion.

## Swiss Ball Pull-In

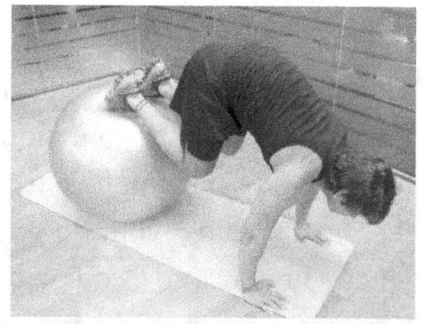

The exercise is somewhat similar to rollouts, requiring your lower abdominals to contract isometrically, stabilizing your spine. In a push-up position with the Swiss ball under your knees and feet, roll the ball towards you. Your knees will come away from the ball and your feet will do the work. Return to the start position and repeat.

## Cycle Crunch

Lie flat on the floor with your lower back pressed to the ground. Put your hands beside your head. Bring your knees up to about a 45-degree angle and slowly go through a bicycle pedal motion. Touch your left elbow to your right knee, then your right elbow to your left knee. Breath evenly throughout the exercise.

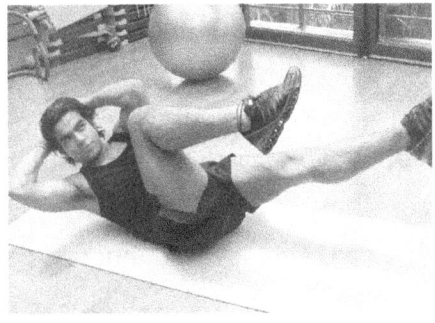

## Bent Knee Bridge

Lie on your back with your knees bent. Place your heels on top of the ball. Lay with your arms spread either side of you. Lift your butt off the floor while squeezing it and push your hips upwards toward the ceiling. Hold at the top and then lower back down to the starting position.

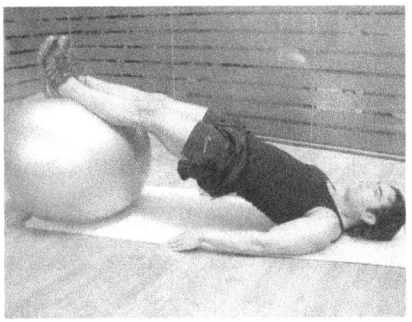

## Medicine Ball Reverse Curls

Lie with your back on the floor or bench with hips flexed at 90° and your feet in the air holding onto a medicine ball between your knees. Position your arms at your sides with palms down on the floor. Leading with the heels towards the ceiling, raise your glutes (butt) off the floor. Return to the start position and repeat. Remember to keep your legs from swinging to prevent momentum throughout the exercise. You may cross your feet together as shown in the photograph.

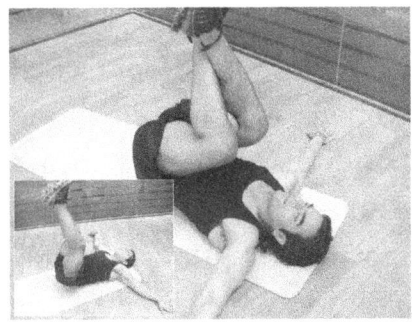

## Leg Pushaway

With your hips and knees bent to 90 degrees. Place your hands under your lower back and press down so that you feel the pressure of your lower back on your hands. Try and slowly lower one leg to touch the ground and return it to the start position whilst maintaining

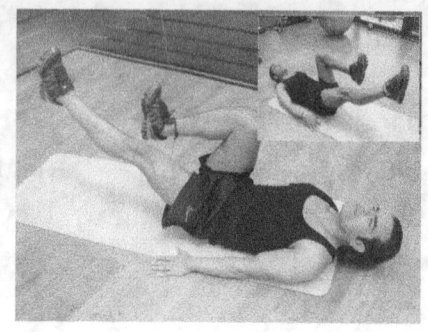

pressure on the hands. Repeat with the other leg.

## Decline on Bench *Optional Exercise

Using a decline bench, lie on your back with your head at the top of the bench, near where your feet usually go. Next, hold the top of the bench with both hands. Hold your legs straight out together in the air, parallel to the floor using your abs to hold them there. Slowly bring your pelvis up and in towards your chest, having your abs control the movement. Slowly lower yourself back to the starting position, always keeping constant tension on your midsection.

## Hanging Leg Raises    Neil's Favorite

Use an overhand grip and grab onto the bar, while keeping your body in a straight line. Keeping your upper body still, lift your legs out in front of you. Hold briefly at the top of the motion, and then slowly lower to the starting position. *Tips:* Move in a slow and controlled manner so that momentum does not take over. Moving in a slow and controlled manner will also decrease how much you will sway. Keep a

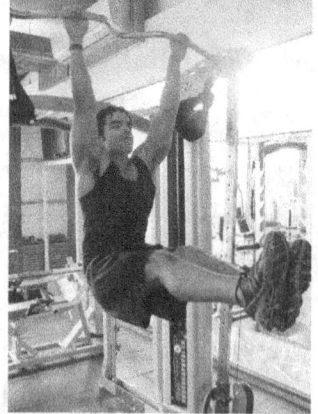

slight bend in the knees to take a little pressure off your lower back. If your grip strength prevents you from holding yourself up, you can use straps to suspend your body

# Hand Positioning

You can increase the level of difficulty to exercises by simply using various hand positioning.

### Hands Above Head

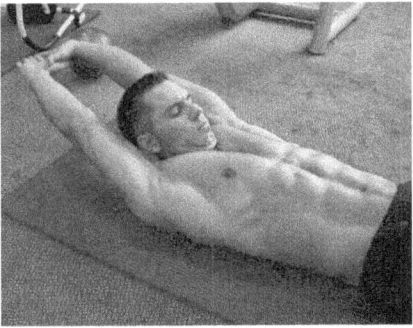

### Hand by Side

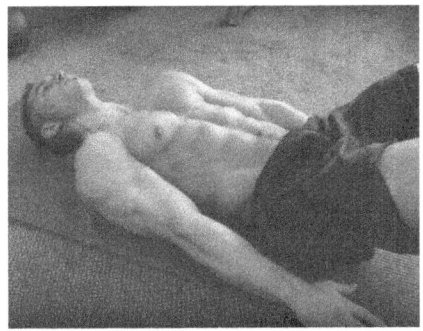

### Hands Behind Head

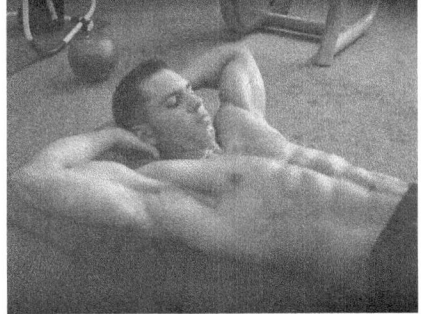

### Hands over Chest

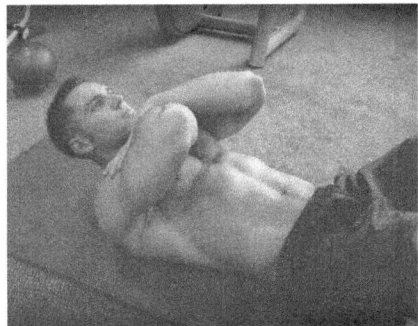

### Hands by Side

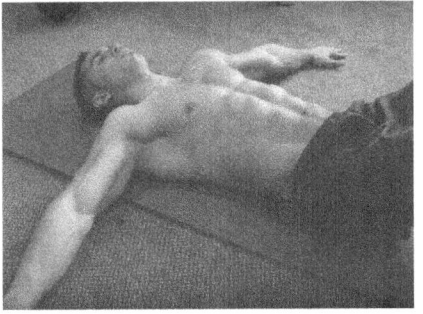

# Advice & Information

In this chapter you'll learn some interesting facts that will help you build your best body.

- **Breaking a Plateau**

- **Abs Top Ten**

- **Water Intake – The Benefits**

- **Hardcore Abs Session**

- **Advanced Cutting Technique**

- **Sugar – The No.1 Culprit for adding fat!**

- **Q & A Section – Nutrition**

- **Q & A Section – Exercise**

- **Q & Section – The Program**

# Breaking A Plateau

**Break a plateau with these simple methods**

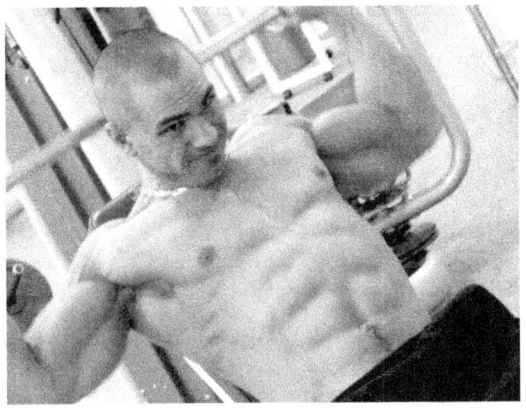

When you first start exercising with weights, you gain muscle mass relatively quickly because of the initial growth spurts from the new shock to your muscles, but after time the results gradually slow. If you have been training for a while, you know I'm talking about what every trainee dreads, reaching a plateau!

Once you reach a plateau, it seems nothing will help you break though it. But there is hope! In fact, there is more than one hope: there are *plateau-breakers*.

If you've been training for years, then you'll know all about them. You've heard the rumours and the myths; you've heard countless guys at the gym claim they have the best plateau-breaker. But which one is the best? What techniques can help me get back to making gains? Here is a run-down of the best plateau-breakers to get your body, building muscle once again. It should be remembered that trainees are encouraged to change their exercise routines every five weeks to avoid reaching a plateau in the first place.

## Exercise Rotation

This is a very simple principle and it works very effectively. Stick to your routine for a few weeks, then, instead of changing your entire program, simply rotate the order in which you usually perform your exercises.

Let's say you train your biceps with three different exercises in which you start with a dumbbell curls, then preacher curls and finish off with cable curls. Rotating exercises will involve putting the cable curls in first place and the dumbbell curls third.

Once you rotate exercises, your second exercise should keep the same weight used as when it was in first position. It will feel heavier, since you will be doing it second, but you will be able to handle it.

Finally, a few weeks later, you should change back and put dumbbell curls first again. Having gotten used to the old weight while doing the exercise second, doing it first should be effortless. And since it will be effortless, you should be able to add more weight. Hey Presto! You have broken through your plateau. This is the best plateau-breaker and it doesn't get any simpler or more effective than this.

## Drop Sets

This principle will shock your body like you never thought possible. Unlike pyramiding (see page 252), instead of adding more weight, decrease the poundage as you go along, while maintaining the same repetitions. Start your exercise the same as always (8-12 reps), but as soon as you are done, reduce the amount of weight and quickly perform another set. Continue doing so until you can't execute a set, even with the smallest amount of weight.

Drop sets are an amazing way of stimulating your muscles, but can be a little impractical as some exercises will require a spotter or an aid because of the amount of weight-changing that's involved. Nevertheless, drop sets rank top amongst the best plateau-breakers.

**Tired of your plateau? There's more you can do...**

Here's one most body-builders and fitness fanatics love: not doing anything! Yes, this is considered a plateau-breaker and a good one too! However, there's more to it than just sitting on the couch all day, but the fundamental principle around this plateau-breaker is resting.

Over-training is a reality in weight training. Too much exercise is unhealthy; the body needs time to heal, recuperate and recover. Sometimes, muscles need a lot of time to heal. If you have been working out for months straight (including those rest days in between cycles), then your body could use a week off every now and then. Yes, a whole week off!

Working out too much for long periods can lead to muscular fatigue. Long rests are like vacations from training and can give the body that much needed re-charge it so needs. Taking a few days or a week off will fill you with a new desire and interest when you do return and you'll find a new growth spurt from this new shock.

## Forced Reps

Forced repetitions are performed by having somebody spot you while you push through a set heavier than you're normally accustomed to doing. Your last reps often end with the spotter helping you out so you can finish your set, which will take on a whole new intensity.

Forced reps are effective; they shock the muscles and can help you break through a plateau, but because of their efficiency, most guys at the gym overuse it. It only works when you have a spotter help you out every now and then..

## Pyramiding

Pyramiding is a very exhaustive technique. It revolves around body building's fundamental principle of adding more weight to each following set. Pyramiding is simply a more extreme variation of this principle.

Start out lifting light (15 reps) then add more weight for each consecutive set. Lower the repetitions for each set since they get heavier. A classic pyramid would look something like this:

15, 12, 10, 8, 6, 4, 2 reps. Each time, add more weight so that you execute each set to failure (i.e. you can't perform another rep).

When you use this method, you usually drop a few exercises from your routine because this single exercise counts for two. It hurts like hell, and by the end you might feel like a fool because you're barely able to make 2 reps. But the sure thing is that it's going to make you grow.

**Partials**

This one's a classic Joe Weider principle which was used by the Great Arnold Schwarzenegger himself; when lifting weights, every now and then you'll reach a sticking point. A sticking point is when you can't lift any more despite the fact that you are not feeling a burn or fatigue. Your muscle still has the energy, but it just doesn't want to move - it just sticks there.

The theory, and the barrier-breaking principle behind it, is to keep lifting even if you can't make a full repetition. If your body wants to stick at a certain point, give it what it wants but keep pushing yourself until you finish your desired amount of reps. If it means only lifting halfway, then that's what you will do, hence the name *partials*.

I'm not done just yet, there's plenty more to choose from...

All exercises are divided into two parts: a positive and a negative motion. When bench-pressing, for example, lifting the barbell is a positive motion and lowering the bar is a negative one. Negative motions are important in body-building. A lot of people don't know that the pain felt the next day comes mainly from the negative part of an exercise done the previous day.

Negatives strengthen your tendons and force your stabilizers (supportive muscles) to work harder. This technique will stimulate growth and help performance. To do a negative properly, you should always lower the weight slowly. Sometimes you can add an extra set to your exercise doing only negatives (a spotter will be needed).

**Rest Pause**

Trust me, you're going to hate this one! Because I certainly do, but it does work wonders when thrown in every once in a while. Okay, it's not that bad, but it is a painful principle and it doesn't directly make your muscles grow.

Lifting 85 to 90% of your one rep maximum (the amount of weight you can lift only once), do 3 reps and rest for 30 seconds. Then lift the same weight again for 2-3 reps and rest for 45 seconds. Then do 2 reps and rest for 60. Lift 1-2 reps, rest for 90 seconds and finish it off with 1 repetition.

That was your first set... You now have two more to go.

There are different variations of this principle, but this one makes the most sense since you get more time to rest as you go along. It works but Rest-Pause, despite being used in body-building, is more of a strength training exercise than a mass-inducing principle. You might gain mass, but in general it will affect your strength and endurance more.

**Compound Sets**

Also know as the "Super-Set," is a compound set in which you perform two exercises for the same body part, one after the other, with no rest in between.

A classic example of a compound set is the Tricep Press/Tricep Extension exercise. While lying down on a flat bench, using an E-Z bar or dumbbells, do tricep presses by pushing the weight upward, as if you were pushing away from a wall. When you finish that set, immediately perform extensions by lowering the weight(s) to your head, moving only your forearms while keeping the rest of the arm still and perpendicular to the floor.

Compound sets are quite effective, but there are few exercises that allow such combinations. Time is of the essence because you need to perform both exercises uninterruptedly.

## Changing Routines

Let us start with the basics. Changing routines every month and a half is the most frequently used method to shock muscles, and for good reason because it works. The body has a tendency to get used to things, so keeping it on its toes is sometimes all you need to get results.

You can change a routine by simply using different exercises, or you can change the weight. Modifying exercises is simple: you use different exercises. That actually goes without saying; every body-builder should do this, no ifs or buts about it. Changing the weight means going from a heavy routine (8-10 reps) to a light routine (12-15 reps). Both variations will give you results.

## Keep the effect

These are the top plateau-breakers. Remember, physique development is not a perfect science and what works for one person might not work for another.

Keep in mind that gimmicks are nice, but sticking to basics usually works best in muscle building. If you do decide to use any "plateau-breaker," do not overuse it because it will lose its effect. Have fun and try some of those plateau-breakers out.

# Tips for Definition

### 1 - Lower Abs

Building the upper abs is relatively easy once your fat layer has been reduced, since almost every ab motion involves a contraction of the upper region. The majority of ab exercises work the upper abs at the cost and neglect of the lower abs. Meanwhile, even exclusive training of the lower abs will still result in impressive upper-ab development.

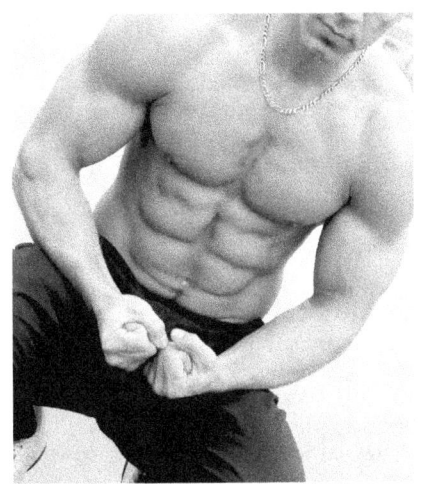

### 2 - Reverse Crunch and Variations

Undoubtedly doing variations of reverse crunches is the most effective way to train your abs. By flexing the hip and rotating the legs, you engage so much more muscle. They do so much for functional strength because they demand that you use the entire anterior core to propel your legs up and knees toward your chest. Rotating the legs both inward and outward add a critical variation. This motion holds the key to good midsection development as it stresses the bulk of the central muscle of the abdomen with an emphasis on the lower area.

### 3 - Don't rep yourself into oblivion

Frequently people go crazy with repetitions, doing dozens or even hundreds per set. After a certain point you stop stimulating and start annihilating. Overuse of these muscles in such sequence can lead to over-training and injuries like the common epigastric hernia (a tear in the tissue in the center of the abdomen that connects the two sides of the rectus abdominis called the linea alba). Granted, abs do require a slightly higher rep scheme than your average body part. However, I tend to keep my reps around 20-30 (fatigue point) or less while instead increasing the level of difficulty with either added resistance or a steeper bench angle if I find I can perform more than 40 reps easily.

## 4 - Don't do too much weighted twisting

While twisting motions might seem like a great way to warm up or start your abs routine, they're actually quite dangerous if you twist too much with weight. For example, holding a barbell across your back and twisting can expose the lumbar spine to disc injury (the worst is in the seated position). Just stick to the basics, a stick or just the barbell bar would be good.

## 5 - Slim Waist? Avoid Heavy Weighted Side-bends

The abdominal muscles, like other muscles in your body, will grow with the stimulus of resistance training. If your goal is a small waist, you don't want to overdevelop muscles that will give you a wider appearance. Unfortunately, doing dumbbell side bends with a very heavy weight will do just that, stimulating the muscles of the external obliques, located in the lower outer abdominal region. When excessively stimulated by resistance training, these muscles can grow and make your waist look wide and blocky, so if you don't want an overly muscular stomach stick with light weighted side bends, not heavy.

## 6 - Squeeze and Flex your Abs

One of the big mistakes you can make with abdominal training is not to flex the muscles as you train them. Too many people just go through the movements without squeezing hard. They view the ab session as an afterthought where they can just coast there way through it. Provide the same attention as you would with any other body part you want to develop.

## 7 - Maintain a slow descent

As with any other exercise, your descent should be slow and controlled, relative to your faster concentric (positive) motion. This is the key when attempting to dig deep into the fibers of the abs and really sculpt them.

## 8 - Don't do forced reps or negatives if a beginner to ab exercising

These advanced training principles will only work for experienced trainees. If you're a beginner do not be tempted to jump straight in and go to failure, its overkill. You will gain no added benefit to having a partner help you through forced reps or resistance-based negative ab training whilst still a beginner to ab work. Implementing such tactics will give you no edge and is almost a certain way to get injured in the early stages of your program. Gradually build up your endurance over the coming weeks.

## 9 - Train your abs with more intensity but less frequency

Too often many fitness freaks train their abs every day. They tend to forget that the abdominals are just like other muscles, in that they need rest to recuperate and improve. Although the abs can be exposed to a bit more frequency in terms of the number of times you train them in a week when compared to other body parts, training them more than three times each week is excessive and overkill, it will not speed up results by doing more!

## 10 - Whenever possible, get a partner to train abs with you

Ab training gets a little monotonous. Because the rep scheme is higher, training frequency is greater and you use no or very little resistance, your effort and intensity level can naturally get a little flat. You can avoid this unpleasant situation by grabbing a partner who has the same goals with you and run through the abs workout with them. This makes it more fun and a healthy competition between you and your partner can boost your intensity.

# Benefits of Water!

**Accelerate fat loss, reduce water retention, increase your performance and improve your physique....with water!**

I'm sure you've heard it many a times before, that drinking more water provides a multitude of benefits to a healthy body. Yes, it may be bland, boring and tasteless, but when I tell you just how drinking **6-8 glasses of water** a day can help you build muscle, accelerate fat loss and reduce water retention, you may just take my advice and drink more of it.

Much emphasis is placed on intaking enough protein, carbs and essential fatty acids, macronutrient ratios and high performance supplements, it's little wonder that something as simple as good old $H_2O$ (Water) could be so easily taken for granted. I cannot emphasize enough the importance of drinking plenty of water and keeping adequately hydrated each day.

Believe it or not, water occupies approximately 60-70% of your body. Your blood is made up of about 90% water. Your muscles are about 70% . Even your bones are 20% water therefore, without adequate water, nothing in your body could function efficiently and operate at optimal levels. Studies show that we lose approximately 1 liter of water a day through our skin and lungs and this amount can be increased dramatically if working out on a regular basis. Therefore, it is essential to replace this loss.

### Dehydration and its effects on physical performance

As you become dehydrated through lack of water, your body's core temperature increases. This adversely affects your cardiovascular function and reduces your capacity for physically demanding work and this includes working out. Even a small decrease in your body's hydration level can decrease your performance. Studies have shown that even mild dehydration can decrease strength by 10%.

### Higher protein diets require higher water intake levels

Because this program tends to be moderate to high in protein, drinking plenty of water is especially important. Not only to keep you hydrated as mentioned above, but to keep bodily functions working properly. With the higher protein intake when the body processes protein it generates metabolic waste products that must be flushed out and removed by the kidneys. Without adequate water, the kidneys can't remove these wastes efficiently. There is a well known myth that high protein diets cause kidney damage. Let me inform you, a high protein diet is not harmful to healthy kidneys -- as long as plenty of water is consumed daily.

### Water is essential to burning fat

Yes, drinking more water increases fat loss! As mentioned above one of the important functions of your kidneys is to eliminate waste products from your body through the urine. When you're dehydrated, the body's instinctive reaction is to hold on to whatever water it does have in order to survive. When this water retention occurs, the waste products in the body aren't flushed out, and build up in your system. At this point, the liver will try to help out with the overload. The problem is, when the liver helps out during fluid retention, it can't do its own jobs as efficiently, one of which is burning stored body fat for energy. The result is that your body may not be able to burn body fat as efficiently as normal. Water is the most valuable aspect of a healthy diet. It's responsible for thousands of biochemical reactions at the cellular level inside the body and also works as an anti-catabolic substance as it eliminates dehydration which of course can be extremely catabolic to muscle tissue. Last but not least according to some latest researches, water has a thermogenic effect. In fact by drinking ice-cold water metabolism is boosted by 30% to bring the temperature up to normal body temperature.

## Drinking more water will help eliminate water retention

Many people avoid drinking a lot of water because they think it will make them retain fluid and become bloated. Actually, the opposite is true. Drinking an adequate amount of water every day is the best treatment for fluid retention, however, if you're dehydrated it perceives the shortage as a threat to survival and will begin to retain every drop present in the body. The best way to overcome the problem of water retention is to give your body what it needs, plenty of water! Only then will stored water be released. Water retention shows up as a layer of water between the skin and muscle resulting in a bloated appearance, hiding any muscle definition which can sometimes be more noticeable around the stomach, face and legs. If you pinch an inch of skin on your stomach, can you feel gristle? No? Then this confirms you have water retention and need to drink more water. If you can feel a gristle like texture then this also confirms that you have excess body fat.

If water retention is a constant problem for you it may be that an intake of excess salt may be to blame. Your body can only tolerate sodium in certain concentrations. The more salt you eat, the more water your system retains to dilute it. But the solution to eradicating this is very simple, just drink more water!

### Don't rely on your level of thirst and a hydration indicator

Your level of thirst is never a good indicator of your level of hydration. By the time your body registers the sensation of thirst, you're already somewhat dehydrated. Therefore, you should continue drinking water throughout the day, even when you're not thirsty. The secret is not to let yourself get dehydrated in the first place. If in doubt, drink more, not less.

### Drink water before, during and after your workout

You should make it a habit to drink water all day long, but because water is so important for energy production and because exercise dehydrates you, you should make it a habit to drink heavily before, during and after your workout.

### Can I get my fluids from other sources?

Almost all of the foods you eat contain water. Some foods, such as fruits and vegetables are as much as 75 to 90 percent water. Even meat is at least 50% water. Other beverages such as milk, fruit juice and sports drinks are mostly water. The question is, should you count these towards your daily recommended intake of water or not? Some sports nutritionists say yes, you can and should count water rich foods towards your water intake. My suggestion is to always err on the side of too much water rather than too little.

## What else can I drink?

On a fat burning program, it's never a good idea to drink a large portion of your calories. One reason is because liquids don't have the thermic effect that solid food does. If you carefully count your liquid calories (juice, sports drinks, non-fat milk or beverages) into your daily calorie allotment, there's no reason you can't enjoy these beverages. Be very careful to read the labels on all beverages you consume, especially sports drinks. Some sports nutrition products that are marketed as high performance health foods" are nothing more than sugar water. Even well-formulated products haven't been proven to increase performance in athletes. For workouts lasting less than an hour, water is still the best thing you can drink. For fat loss purposes, why would you want all those extra simple carbohydrates anyway?

## What about diet drinks and non-caloric drinks?

As long as you're getting your daily allotment of pure water, it's fine to enjoy non-caloric beverages such as diet soda, tea, coca-cola light or any other calorie free/sugar free diet drinks. Coffee is also fine in moderation (one or two cups per day), but be careful what you put in it. (We're talking regular black coffee here with maybe a splash of skimmed milk – no sugar). Enjoy your coffee in moderation – a cup or two per day should pose no problem. Keep in mind that caffeine is a diuretic and large amounts of any diuretic can decrease your performance and your results.

# SUMMARY:

- Always keep a bottle of water to hand

- Men consuming 175 grams or less of Protein per day should aim for 6-8 x 250ml glasses of water per day.

- Men consuming more than 175 grams of protein per day should aim for 8-10 x 250ml glasses of water per day.

- During particularly hot weather water intake should be inceased

# GOING HARDCORE

A great set of abs is a function of two factors, abdominal muscle density and low body-fat. Having a low body-fat level (below 10% for men and 15% for women) plays a significant role, because the less of it you have the more visible the abs become.

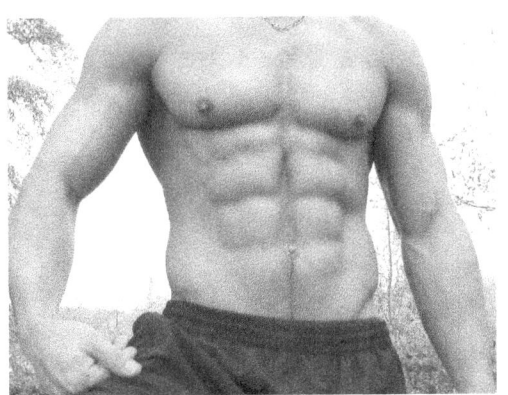

As far as ab exercises go there are literally hundreds I could have shown you in the book, but in all honesty unless you have low enough body fat your abs are not going to show, no matter how much you keep working them. Many ab exercises don't even work the abs sufficiently either apart from those outlined in the Bollywood Abs Workout (Page 227). In fact scientists have an amazing tool called Electromyography (EMG) that shows how much muscles work during specific exercises by placing electrodes over the stomach muscles. The harder the muscle works the more electricity is measured on the EMG. These EMG studies have shown the best ab exercises to be bench crunches, hanging leg raises, cable crunches, swiss ball crunches, vertical crunches (especially on a swiss ball) and swiss ball side crunches.

So let's place these exercises into a hardcore workout. This routine is only for people who have a more advanced level of experience in doing ab exercises with proper form and have a body fat percentage under 15%.

The workout will involve 4 giant-sets including all of the exercises mentioned above, with 1 minute rest between them in order to keep the heart rate high. A giant-set is a very intensive set that consists of various exercises with very little rest in-between. Only when you perform this whole series of exercises can you rest a little according to your fitness level. So here it is:

## GIANT-SET:

1) Bench Crunches X max reps

2) Hanging Leg Raises X max reps

3) Cable Crunches X max reps

4) Swiss Ball Crunches X max reps

5) Swiss Ball Vertical Crunches X max reps

6) Swiss Ball Side Crunches X max reps

As you can see half of the ab routine includes swiss ball exercises. Using the ball you can work through a greater range of motion, activate more muscle fibers than regular exercises and therefore make more intensive ab workouts when performed properly. Now let's take a look at each exercise alone.

1) **Bench Crunches:** Lie flat on the floor with the legs over a bench so that the thighs are perpendicular to the floor. Cross the arms over the chest. Once you are in the proper starting position, simply raises your upper back off the floor very slowly and roll forward until you reach the end point of the movement.

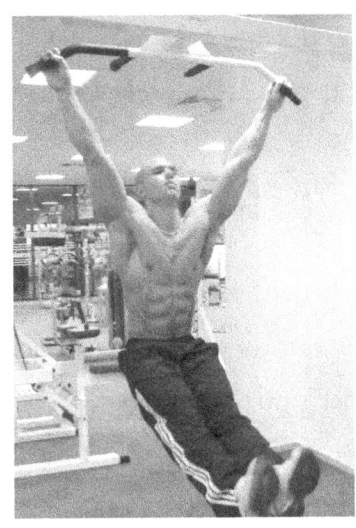

2) **Hanging Leg Raises:** Take an overhand grip on a pull-up bar with your hands about shoulder-width apart and allow your body to hang freely without your feet touching the floor. Keeping your legs straight and toes pointed, exhale and slowly lift your legs upward, avoiding the use of momentum until your body forms an "L" shape in mid-air. Pause a moment before slowly lowering your legs back to the start.

3) **Cable Crunches:** Use the rope attachment on the high cable pulley. Kneel facing the machine and grasp the rope and put your hands against your forehead. Lock your arms to your head so that you are using your abs to pull the weight not your arms.

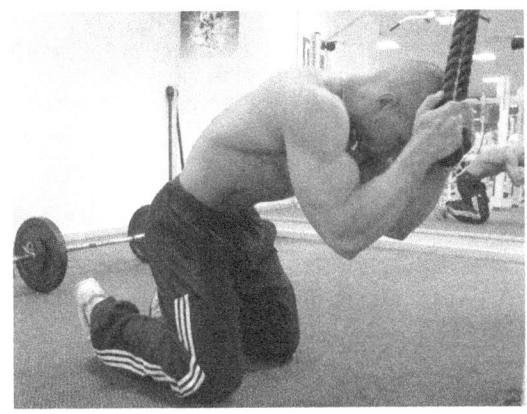

You then begin the exercise by slowly moving your body downwards in an arc, rounding your back and trying to get your elbows to touch your knees. Contract for 2 seconds hard before returning to the starting position.

4) **Swiss Ball Crunches:** Balance yourself on an exercise ball with your arms folded across your chest, focus your eyes on the ceiling with your feet flat on the floor. Your starting position should find your back slightly arched over the curve of the ball. Exhale and slowly lift your upper body

off the ball, keeping your focus high and your elbows wide. Pause a moment in the topmost position before inhaling and slowly lowering yourself back to the start.

5) **Swiss Ball Vertical Crunches:** Position a bench near the swiss ball so you be able to grasp it. Lie on the ball with your hands over your head gripping the bench behind it, your back flat and your knees bent and held above your hips. This is your starting position. From here, slowly curl your knees up and in toward your head, lifting first your tailbone, then your hips, off the ball. When your knees come to eye level, reverse the motion and slowly uncurl. Pass the start position and extend your legs straight out and away from you, keeping your back stable on the ball and your shoulders down. Squeeze for a moment and come back to the starting position.

6) **Swiss Ball Side Crunches:** Lie sideways on a swiss ball, place your feet on the floor, knees bent and spread your legs so your feet are slightly more than shoulder width apart. Slowly raise your upper and mid back off the ball and turn to your right so you are in an oblique curl position. Squeeze for a second and then slowly return to the starting position.

# Advanced Cutting Technique

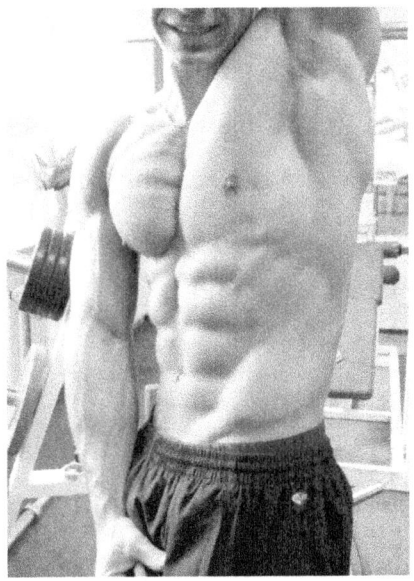

What diets do fitness models and bodybuilders use to get that shredded look? Are there any advanced techniques to get really cut like these guys?

Yes there are, but I must stress, this is for **advanced trainees only**. It would be pointless using this cutting method if you're not experienced with both dieting and weight training. This will also only work with someone with substantial muscle mass. The technique below is used by competitive bodybuilders and fitness models to prepare their bodies for stage/photo condition.

You only have to look at competitive bodybuilders and fitness models these days to see how lean and shredded they can get. The pictures you see of guys on the magazines with their onion tight skin condition and single digit body fat percentage has every muscle fiber and striated tissue visible. But how do these guys get like that? Here's a 12 week insight into obtaining ultimate condition without losing too much muscle mass.

A cutting diet will vary from person to person, but usually a bodybuilder will dedicate 12 weeks to get in competition condition, where as a fitness model who would typically be leaner may only need 4-6 weeks. For this example we will take a look at a 12 Week strategy.

By far the hardest part of the cutting up strategy is the diet! The days of eating cheeseburgers and pizza are long gone and the key now is to gradually reduce calories whilst holding on to as much muscle as possible, optimally losing no more than a pound or two a week. Any more weight loss per week will risk you stepping on stage or for a photo shoot looking smaller and flatter from excessive muscle wasting. If you give your body the right amount of nutrients and calories to lose that one to two pounds per week, you will find yourself looking bigger and better naked! Even though your clothes will be a bit baggy on you by the end of your diet.

Here's a look at a cutting diet for a 220 pound individual who would expect to lose approximately 15-25 pounds during this 12 Week Plan:

## INDIAN STYLE NON VEG - HIGH CARB DAY

1. Breakfast Chapati (2 wholewheat chapatis). 1 scoop of whey in water
2. Whey Shake ( 1.5 scoops in water with 2-3 heaped tablespoons of oats)
3. Tandoori Chicken with Rice Dish
4. Whey Shake ( 1.5 scoops in water with 1 piece of fruit)
5. Lean Wholewheat Chapatis with Beef, chicken or turkey (100-125gcooked weight, in 2-3 chapatis)
6. Whey or Casein Protein Shake in water

## INDIAN STYLE NON VEG - HIGH CARB DAY

1. Egg White Omelette with Tea or Coffee (no sugar)
2. Chicken Chapati – (203 Wholewheat Chapatis)
3. Pineapple Chicken Kebabs
4. Whey Shake ( 1.5 scoops in water with 1 piece of fruit)

5. Tuna Curry with 2-3 Wholewheat Chapatis or Dhal/Rice Dish

6. Whey or Casein Protein Shake in water with 10g Glutamine

## WESTERN STYLE - HIGH CARB DAY

1. 06.00 - 8 eggs (1-2 yolks) 1 bowl of oatmeal (enough for about 70 grams of carbs, about 1 cup) and multi-vitamin.

2. 08.30 - Protein shake with 16 oz of with water and omega 3 fatty acid, CLA, or Flax Oil.

3. 10.30 – 1 can of tuna with mustard and 1 Wholegrain Bagel and 5 grams of Glutamine

4. 13.00 - (after workout) Protein shake with Glutamine and yams and Vitamin C/E.

5. 16.00 - 150g of chicken breast, 1-cup brown rice or yam with green veggies

6. 19.00 - 150g of chicken breast or fish (tuna, salmon, or whatever you like) with broccoli or green beans or salad with balsamic vinegar or lemon juice.

7. 21.30 – Lean Sirloin or Flank Steak with salad and balsamic vinegar (eat Steak 2x per week.)

8. Bedtime - 1 scoop of protein and Glutamine in water or 200g of Dry Curd Cottage Cheese

## WESTERN STYLE - LOW CARB DAY

1. 06.00 - 8 eggs (1-2 yolks) 1 bowl of oatmeal (enough for about 40 grams of carbs, about 1/2 cup) and multi-vitamin.

2. 08.30 - Protein shake with 16 oz of with water and omega 3 fatty acid, CLA, or Flax Oil.

3. 10.30 – 1 can of tuna with mustard and 4 rice cakes and 5 grams of Glutamine

4. 13.00 - (after workout) Protein shake with Glutamine and Vitamin C

5. 16.00 - 150g of chicken breast with green veggies

6. 19.00 - 150g of chicken breast or fish (tuna, salmon, or whatever you like) with broccoli or green beans or salad with balsamic vinegar or lemon juice.

7. 21.30 – Lean Sirloin or Flank Steak with salad and balsamic vinegar (eat Steak at least 2x per week.)

8. Bedtime - 1 scoop of protein and Glutamine in water or 200g of Dry Curd Cottage Cheese

The most important part of the cutting diet is cycling carbohydrates throughout the week and using those carbs only when needed. By that I mean using them when you need energy for weight training or cardio. The majority of carbs should be consumed early in the day so that you can burn them off before going to sleep that evening.

After about three days of low carbs, I usually spike it up to have one high carb day to prevent my body from losing muscle mass and energy. I basically start with oatmeal, yams, wholegrain bagels or brown rice with my meals equalling about 150 grams of carbs for the first day, 100 grams the next day, 50 grams the 3rd, then go all the way back up to around 200-250 grams the 4th 'Spike' day. This allows your metabolism to remain high by confusing the body into not getting used to a constant low carb diet, which can play havoc on your mood and memory (a side affect of low carbohydrate dieting).

Also to make the diet less painful, you can still allow certain seasoning on foods to include mustard, salt, pepper, and garlic and of course all Indian spices. This only changes the last week before the show or photo shoot, which is the most important time during the dieting phase. The last ten days can make or break you when it comes to achieving peak condition.

Ten days prior to the event, the major changes I make in my diet are the manipulation of my water, sodium and potassium. If done correctly, you can shed a good 3-5% body fat in those 10 days. This process will make your skin so paper thin that you will look like an anatomy chart and be one of the leanest athletes for competition or photos.

First, ten days prior I add more sodium than I usually had during my normal 8-12 week diet. Usually I just add more salt to my boiled eggs, chicken and steak, and eat a lot more fish. Don't be afraid that this extra sodium will bloat you or blur your condition, this is where your extra water consumption will help you. During the preparation period, I usually consume just under 4 liters of water a day. During my ten day manipulation phase, I increase my water to 5-6 liters. This will trick your body into getting rid of water and it will also flush out the excess sodium. Expect frequent visits to the bathroom during this phase. **Please be advised,** water manipulation is an **advanced technique**. For novices I would encourage you to skip the Sodium and Water Manipulation Phase and continue to drink approximately 3 liters daily until 3 days out. You will still get in spectacular condition.

Three days prior to the event, I make another change. I now begin to drop my water and sodium by 1/3 and start to add either potassium pills or dandelion root (which contains potassium in it and works wonders for getting rid of water retention from under the skin). I also switch my water from regular drinking water to Mineral water, some use distilled water. In fact, when you drink the mineral or distilled water, you will not feel bloated like you would with regular water and you will probably feel thirstier, but you will still urinate a lot. I also drop my carbohydrate consumption each day starting on the Monday before the event (which is Saturday in this case) until I hit just 25-50 grams on Wednesday. Two days prior to the show/photoshoot I slowly add more carbs into my diet until the event (Carb Loading). On these days you will increase carbs significantly (250-350g and above) to fill out your muscles. These will be high carb days. At this point you need to keep an eye on your condition as too many carbs will make you bloated, so you can cut back slightly one day prior to the event dependant of course on how you look in the mirror. Two days prior I also reduce the salt and water again, this time getting rid of almost all sodium I possibly can and dropping my water down to only one gallon (4.5 Liters). The day before the event, once again no sodium and drink about a half a gallon (2 Liters) of mineral or distilled water till around noon, and then just take sips when needed for the dandelion root pills or multi-vitamins. Ice cubes can be used on occasion, but only when really needed. Each day you will literally see and feel your skin tighten and your weight drop and the water from your skin vanish. It is important to pose hard to squeeze out all of the water (I start to practice my posing about one month prior to a competition to build up stage presence and muscular endurance) and to tan a few weeks prior to also draw water from out of your skin as well, but don't use tanning booths 3-4 days before the event to allow your skin to heal from possible burning from the booths. Artificial tanning lotions are recommended during the last few days to give your skin a healthy, toned look that enhances definition for the stage and photos. The day before the show/shoot is pretty much the same as the previous day, however, watching your condition is very important as you can easily carb overload, so keep checking yourself, making sure your stomach is not bloated. If you're ok, then continue with dry oats, rice cakes or sweet potatoes with your meals. The night before the contest I have a 150g fillet steak or turkey with 150g of baked potato. If I still feel I've not filled out then I continue to eat some dry oats (40g in weight) every hour or two.

On the day of the Contest/Shoot I start the day with a meal of 150g Steak and 200g of Baked Potato. Assuming the contest or shoot is at 1pm I will continue sipping water only when really needed. From then on protein is not really needed, I concentrate on keeping my muscles full with carbs like 30g of dry oats and 2-3 rice cakes every hour until the event. Two hours before I add a tablespoon or two of honey and natural peanut butter to my rice cakes and then 30 minutes before the event I add some raisins and a couple of chunks of dark chocolate along with a small pot of flavoured jelly. This sugar gets the vascularity out and is where the competition condition really sets in. I have a five minute pump up with some free weights or resistance bands, just before going on stage or having my photo taken, this really gets your muscles pumped and ready. A little oil can now be rubbed on to your body to make the final touch.

For pre-contest training, my weight training consists of hitting each body part once a week except my weak body parts (shoulders, upper chest and back) which I train along with other muscle groups briefly when I can fit them in (I usually save one day on the weekend to train all three at once). I slowly increase my tempo during the workouts (less rest between sets) and intensity by adding supersets and drop sets (starting a heavy set of an exercise and either dropping to a lighter weight or another exercise without rest). This is effective for me because I keep my heart rate up and really burn the muscle quickly and I still start with the heavy compound exercises with heavy weight in the beginning to prevent my muscles from shrinking (to me, big weights will always equal big muscles). My training will cease three days before the event, this will allow me the time needed to carb load. For Cardio, I switch to low intensity five days per week as I can't afford to burn any hard earned muscle with higher intensity training. Great workouts include the rotating stair climber, elliptical or stationery bike. I will do cardio upon waking up for 30 minutes. I will also do cardio at night for 20 to 30 minutes, depending on what shape I'm in and how far out of condition I feel I am. This will be performed right after weight training. Constant monitoring of your body is the key to success and you need to be honest and subjective if you want to be the best! Cardio will cease two days before the event.

I advise you **not** to stay on the low sodium and water portion of the diet for an extended period of time. Sodium is vital to many bodily functions and aids in performance, and without it you can suffer serious cramps and discomfort. I also advise you not to go without water for more than a day as serious dehydration can land you in the hospital! In fact, if you are not competing in a contest, I would continue to drink the water right up until the photo shoot, you will still look great and be shredded! If you follow these rules, you will be amazed at how quickly your body will transform. It may take you a while to find out which formula works best for you (some may have to drop there sodium and water sooner or later and manipulate your carbohydrates differently as well), but you will see a difference. Each time you go to the bathroom and urinate, you will literally see and feel your skin get tighter. Water manipulation can be the difference between 3rd and 1st place and for models it can be the difference between being in a magazine article and being on the cover of the magazine!

**Please Note.** Pre-Contest dieting is both physically, mentally and emotionally draining. This hardcore approach challenges you in every way possible and it takes an extremely dedicated trainee to see this through to its end. During this time social events will need to be put to one side, you have to concentrate fully on your goal and keep your mindset focused as you cannot afford to let anything side track you. An understanding partner and positive friends will go a long way in helping you through the ups and downs of this dieting phase. The ultimate goal is one that you can treasure for the rest of your life, so make sure to get your pictures taken!!

# Q & A Section

**Is sugar really that bad for fat loss?**  It's not sugar itself that is unhealthy, it's how we use it and in some cases, abuse it. First of all, sugar is a natural carbohydrate and is found in most fruits and vegetables. Sugar is almost always associated with non-nutritional food like soda pop, candy, and cakes. Have you ever tasted a cake without sugar? It just doesn't taste good so it's necessary to add sugar, therefore, sugar is the one to blame for us getting fat. So how much sugar is really added to that cola you just drank? How about a whopping 40 grams of sugar! - that is equal to 10 teaspoons which equals 150 calories! That is just one twelve ounce can. Try a 16 ounce triple thick chocolate shake and enjoy 84 grams of sugar - over 20 teaspoons!  My advice is to try and avoid sugar where possible, especially when it comes to table sugar or processed foods with a high sugar content.

**I cannot afford why protein or supplements. Can I still build a great body?** Of course!  However, it does mean that you will be missing out on approximately 80 grams of protein per day without them, therefore, it is important to replace this with whole foods high in protein, such as: Meat or Fish, Eggs, Cottage Cheese, Legumes, Lentils, Tofu, Beans or Soy.

**I don't have time to eat five-six meals day. Will it be ok to consume three?**  I cannot emphasize enough the importance of consuming five - six smaller sized meals per day. Eating these smaller meals more frequently throughout the day will speed up your metabolism, meaning that the food will get absorbed much more quickly than a larger meal would. If you don't have time, supplement with a good quality Whey/Soy Protein shake or bar in-between your other meals.

**I noticed that eggs have a lot of fat. Is this okay?** Egg yolks (yellow part) are the part of the egg which has the high fat and cholesterol content, this is why I only recommend the whites. For every four whites, you may have one yolk.

**I am finding it quite difficult to eat the five/six meals per day because I don't feel hungry, but I eat because the program says I should. I was wondering if I am wrong in eating when I'm not hungry, or is that the whole point (to prevent hunger)?** As briefly explained above, eating five or six meals per day is an essential part of any fat loss nutrition plan. The importance is to keep your metabolism rate as high as possible. If people go too long without eating, they tend to overcompensate at the end of the day. It could be that your portions are too big or contain too many carbohydrates hence why they're filling you up too much. As mentioned above my advice would be to supplement with a Protein shake or Meal Replacement Powder mid morning and mid afternoon to act as two meal replacements, this way you don't need to worry about eating a meal. A shake will provide you with all the essential nutrients you need. Your meal plan could look similar to this: 8am: Meal, 10.30: Protein Shake or MRP, 12.30: Meal 3.00: Protein Shake, 5.30: Meal, 8.00: Meal or Shake

**I was just wondering whether or not it is ok to consume alcoholic beverages (mainly beer) while on the program?** Ideally you do need to stay away from alcohol, especially beer. Beer contains a considerable amount of 'empty calories' which your body finds very hard to burn off. It also dehydrates you which causes negative effects on your muscle building potential. You know how a hangover makes you feel, well dehydration is what causes the nastier side effects such as headache, nausea and zero energy. If you really want to look good alcohol (especially beer) must be cut back. Red wine, Whisky or Vodka are much preferred as their calorie content is much lower, however, these drinks are more prone to give hangovers. Drinking once a week is fine, however binge drinking or heavy weekend drinking will ruin progress. If you are out for a special occasion my own personal way to limit a hangover is to try and drink water towards the end of the night in between your beers or other alcoholic drinks. Before bedtime have another full glass of water along with 1-2 slices of bread. This will help soak up the alcohol.

**I am vegan. I do not consume any animal products whatsoever. I really want great muscle definition and I understand that diet is key. My main source of protein is in soy products. My question is, how do I maintain a proper high-protein, low fat diet without compromising my morals?** For the vegan trainee, a strict regimen will need to be followed, to ensure that a varied diet is still consumed. Remember that many quality supplements are derived from animal products, for example whey protein and meal replacement powders (MRPs), so you will have to avoid these. If you are in doubt about any product, check with the manufacturer. As there are so many exclusions in the vegan diet, I strongly feel that isolated soya protein is an absolute must for the vegan trainee in order to meet protein requirements. Other great protein sources which vegetarians and vegans can enjoy are mixed beans, baked beans, vegetables, hummus, tofu, quorn, textured vegetable protein (TVP), nuts and seeds, soya, oat and rice milk, and many more. Rest assured being vegan will not have a negative impact on your success, however self discipline will be called for.

**I'm Lactose Intolerant, can you guide me on some Lactose Free or Low Lactose whey supplements?** Lactose Intolerance is the term used for people who cannot digest dairy products. At birth they were born without a digestive enzyme enabling them to digest most milk and dairy products containing lactose.

Lactose is the ingredient in foods which affects the lactose intolerant negatively. It is found in milk and milk products like cheese and yogurt and also many whey protein supplements. However, many supplement manufacturers use an advanced filtration method that takes out impurities and leaves the powder lactose free.

Currently there are many to choose from, my top five picks would be: Natures Best Isopure, CytoSport CytoGainer, CytoSport MuscleMilk Light, Dymatize ISO-100 and Optimum 100% Whey Gold Standard. Fat Free Soy Milk or water would be best to mix with your powder.

For those who have use or have used regular whey supplements in the past and have felt nauseous, had an upset stomach or felt unusually bloated/gassy it may be worth visiting your doctor as you may have an intolerance to Lactose.

**Is it true what they say about celery? Do you actually burn more calories eating it than you gain from it? If so why not just carry it around and eat it whenever you get the chance? (as an extra to your current diet)** Although celery does not speed up your metabolism, it is actually a negative calorie food - it provides so little nutrients and calories that you burn more energy chewing and digesting it than you gain by metabolising it. Lettuce is another example of a negative calorie food. Here is a list of foods considered 'negative calorie': Asparagus, Broccoli, Cabbage, Carrot, Cauliflower, Celery, Chicory, Hot Chili, Cucumber, Garden cress, Garlic, Green Beans, Lettuce, Onion, Radish Spinach, Zuccini/Courgette

**Is it ok to eat soups?** Ideally you should avoid tinned or packet soup due to the sodium and other additives associated with them, however now and again they are fine. I would particularly recommend making your own Vegetable Soup which will be a much more nutritious and healthier option, here's how to make it: 1 can V-8 juice, 1 can tomatoes, 2 cans mixed vegetables (add juice from cans), 1 pack frozen mix of chopped onion, bell pepper and celery, 1 can new potatoes Season to taste and combine ingredients. Then, cook all day in a crock pot or simmer for about one and a half hours. Alternately if you have a blender, blend up some various vegetables and blend to a pulp and then heat up, simple!

**I've recently lost 70 pounds and I am now at 215 lbs. I don't really want to lose any more weight if at all possible, but I do want a six pack. I was just wondering if there was a way to minimize body fat and obtain a six pack without losing weight in poundage?** You have to remember that 1 pound of fat weighs 1 pound, so if you still have 15 pounds of unwanted fat on your body you will have to lose 15 pounds in weight. However you can balance this out my adding more muscle. As you lose the fat you will also be building new muscle which will allow your weight to even out. Stick to a high protein diet along with hard training and you will maintain your current weight (give or take a few pounds) yet still drop the fat. It's all about finding a happy medium between your diet and right amount of exercise.

**How about consuming egg beaters, as opposed to egg whites? Also I used to mix a big bowl of tuna/brown rice/mustard/tabasco and consume small portions through the day. Is this acceptable?**

Egg Beaters are great, you may want to scramble these or make an omelette, here is a good omelette recipe: 3/4 cup Eggbeaters diced onion, diced peppers (red & green), sliced grape tomatoes, broccoli (just the very tip tops of the floret) Mix it all together in a measuring cup and pour it into a lightly oiled non-stick skillet over low heat. As it firms up after 5min I use pepper and a couple splashes of Tabasco and you have a great omelette. Anything with Tuna is good, the tabasco and mustard will also flavor it up and the brown rice is a 'good carb' so this is fine.

**I've been told that white rice makes you fat. Is that true?** Yes, this is true. White Rice is a highly processed carbohydrate - high on the glycemic index, low in fiber, low in nutrients, and not terribly filling. Eating white rice will massively spike insulin release in the body and leave you feeling hungry again shortly after you eat it. You don't need to go aggressively low-carb to lose fat, but you do want to limit your intake of processed carbs like white rice. White Rice after a hard training session is fine, but your ideal choices are vegetables, brown rice or pasta, sweet potatoes and oatmeal as your primary sources of carbohydrates.

**I've been trying to find good meats to eat, but many have some amount of sodium. How much sodium is too much?** The amounts found in fresh cuts of meat are generally quite low. You'll only see much higher amounts of sodium (salt) in processed meats or cold deli cuts, those you should try to avoid where possible. You should also avoid adding salt to home cooked meals, a pinch of the Salt Substitute Nu-Salt is fine. Also try vinegar, lemon or spices to help with taste. You must try and keep Sodium (Salt intake) **below 6g for men and 5g for women per day.**

# Q & A - Exercise

**I want really cut abs, how can I get them?** This would require a body fat percentage lower than 8%. Once you have lowered your body fat levels to below this I would suggest you begin using weight with your abdominal exercises. This resistance will place more pressure on the abdominal muscles which in turn will build the abdominals and create deeper etches.

**My upper abdominals are more defined than the lower ones. Why is this?** The Lower Abs are by far the hardest section to develop, mostly due to the accumulation of fat in this area. Most fat actually gets stored in the lower region of your stomach, hence why you often get that overhang with your trousers! It really boils down to your overall body fat percentage and if it's still over that 10% mark, which it will be if you cannot see your lower abs, then you still need to reduce it further. At this point harder ab training won't make much of a difference, it's a question of further tightening your diet and increasing aerobic activity to bring your body fat percentage down to single digits. Water retention may also be a factor (see page 215). If your body fat percentage is giving a reading of less than 10% I would encourage you to incorporate more resistance based exercises for the lowers to help push them out.

**I'm quite slim but just have fat covering my abs. Is spot reduction of fat possible?** Spot reduction is simply the idea that if you work a specific muscle group you will decrease the amount of fat in that area. The most common example of this is that people focus solely on abdominal exercises in an effort to lose fat around their stomach. This is all to no avail, because **it has absolutely no effect on burning fat!**

In reality, there is no such thing as spot reduction. You will never attain a flat stomach just by performing abdominal exercises alone. The reason for this is very simple: a muscle does not own the fat that surrounds it. Crunches or Sit-Ups, for example, will certainly strengthen your abdominal muscles, but relying on them alone will not reduce the layer of fat that is covering the muscles. To lose fat anywhere on your body you need to burn calories by following a program that involves both cardiovascular and weight training, along with a new healthier eating plan. In doing so, you will decrease fat stores throughout your entire body, including the problem areas.

**I am just curious how often I should do my ab exercises. Do you recommend every day? I have talked to many people and have gotten many different answers on how often to do them.** Ideally you should be working your abdominals three times weekly, working the upper abs one day, the lower abs two days later and the side obliques a further two days later. Trainees with a considerable amount of body fat (Above 15% body fat) must realize that to see the benefit of more advanced ab workouts you must reduce your body fat percentage first and foremost. This is not to say that ab exercising at this stage has no place, it does. But remember, ab exercises alone do not sculpt great abs, Nutrition and Fat Burning exercise is the key.

**When doing ab exercises I often find that some of my back muscles get tired way faster than my abs do. The back muscles that get tired are in the lower and middle region of my back.** Far too may people encounter this problem because their lower backs are not trained and under-developed. Having a strong core (lower back) is essential when it comes to properly executing abdominal exercises. There are two exercises that I encourage trainees to make staple in their workout routines and they are Deadlifts and Hyperextensions (Page 116). Developing a stronger core will go a long way in getting more out of your ab workouts.

You should also ensure that your muscles are properly warmed up before beginning your workout. Here are a couple of warm up exercises to begin your ab workouts which will relax the back muscles. Lie on the floor with your back on the ground. Pull your knees up, holding your legs in the pocket behind the knees, and pull your chest up toward the knees gently. This isn't a crunch, but a stretch. Breathe deeply and relax. Repeat that, gradually trying to bring your knees in toward your chest. But don't bounce or strain. Do it about 5-6 times. Lie on the floor with your pelvis against the ground. Push up with your arms, still keeping your stomach on the ground, so you are gently bending your back toward the ceiling. Focus on relaxing the lower back. Hold - again, don't bounce or strain - and then go back down. Repeat that a few times, going just a little more each time, but never straining the lower back. Put a pillow or towel on the floor, and rest your right knee on it. Put your left foot in front of you, so your left knee is bent at a right angle. Now, push your pelvis forward, so you start to feel a stretch in your right quadricep (the front of the right leg). Do that several times, focusing on the stretch, and the slight forward movement of the lower spine. Repeat that with the other leg. Do those stretches before your crunches, and in the evening. If you stretch in the morning, be very very gentle, since the back tends to be tighter and the disks more hydrated at that time. Also, when you do your crunches, your lower back should never leave the ground. Rather, your rib cage should move in toward the pelvic bone, and your lower back should press into the ground, while the shoulders only move a few inches off the floor.

**What does a set consist of and how many? And what does 'to failure' mean?** A 'set' is a number of repetitions completed for an exercise. For example: You may choose to perform crunches and the program asks you to complete 3 sets to failure. This means you will perform the exercises three separate times with as many repetitions as possible. Failure, is where you do not count the number of reps you perform, you just keep going until your muscles fatigue or burn out. It is far more important and productive to perform high quality repetitions than to simply 'make it through' the set. A productive set is a string of productive repetitions, not just a certain 'magic number' of repetitions. Don't aim for 8, 10 or 12 reps, keep going till those abs burn.

**Due to my job I am often away from home and therefore have to rely on a hotel gym for my workouts. Is there anything I can do in my hotel room for a workout instead?** I would recommend buying a set of resistance bands. Resistance bands use elastic or hydraulic resistance and are a portable alternative to free weights for strength training. They take up no room in your luggage, are easy to use and offer a good amount of resistance to really work those muscles.

**Should I perform my ab exercises on an empty stomach after cardio or when I do my weight training?** The best time to perform your exercises is when you have a good amount of energy, either early morning or evening is fine, a particularly good time is before your weights workout, not after, but ensure you always perform your ab exercises on an empty stomach or at least 30-45 minutes after food.

**Is there anything wrong with doing ab exercises when I have some fat, I know it won't show till I lose the fat, but feel like I need to exercise the abs?** If you have a high amount of stomach fat covering your abs then their is little point pushing your ab workouts too hard, your time would be put to better use by concentrating more on cardio, however, a couple of workouts each week will help to begin strengthening your abdominals. It will also help you to become familiar with the exercises so that you can perform each exercise properly as soon as your fat layer has been reduced.

**What's the best way to hold plates for ab weighted exercises? I've heard it can be on the chest, behind your head, or in front of your head. Which is the best way?** There is no better way, as long as you execute the movement properly, where you place the weight will increase the resistance making it harder. Try the various methods and see which works best for you. On your chest is a good place to start as it will eliminate any strain on your neck. Once you've mastered this you can try the more advanced option by placing the weight in front of your head. Personally, I would discourage using a weight behind your head, due to the strain this places on your neck muscles.

**I incorporate weights in a few exercises but how can I put them to use in all the exercises?** You can only use weights with selected exercises like, crunches, sit ups, seated and bench raises, cable crunches, leg raises and vertical crunches. With that being said if you take a look at the various exercises displayed in the book you can add weight to most, whether you hold a loose plate on your chest, or out in front of you, this will work well with most basic exercises.

**How can I measure my body-fat?** Measuring body fat with a set of body fat calipers is the most accurate way to determine fat levels. But it's important to use them correctly. It may be easier and more accurate to have a professional take the measurements for you or buy a set of Calipers and follow the measuring instructions.

# Q & A - The Program

**I've been feeling tired and drained since beginning the program, why is this?** Since beginning the program you have taken on a new lifestyle and a new diet, this change will have certain effects on your body. As explained in the Introduction earlier, it is important not to do too much too soon as it can have the reverse effect. Far too many people in their quest for a better body jump in head first and find they burn out in the first couple of weeks. Your body is not used to this, so you must take time and gradually introduce the program. Diet also plays an important role in energy levels, therefore it is important not to drop your carbohydrates too low or you'll end up feeling drained, irritable and lethargic.

**When is the best time to do my cardiovascular training and should it be performed on an empty stomach?** If possible perform cardio first thing in the morning before breakfast when your metabolism is at its most active and your body is in a fasted state. It is important to consume approximately 15g of Protein thirty minutes before performing cardio. This is to ensure your body does not run the risk of muscle catabolism, where you will burn hard earned muscle. So many people perform cardio on an empty stomach thinking they're going to burn more fat. Not true, muscle is being burned with this. Also supplementing with L-Glutamine before cardio has been proven to minimize muscle catabolism. Another effective time to perform cardio is directly after a weight training workout. The reason for doing this is because during your weight training you deplete your body of glycogen. Once depleted, your body can burn fat more efficiently.

**Why HIIT Cardio, can't I just do regular cardio?** Of course, you can implement any of the cardio workouts I mentioned earlier, however, if your main priority is solely fat loss then HIIT is the preferred choice. HIIT Cardio is a very effective cardio workout that cuts regular cardio sessions by half, yet provides great results in terms of fat loss. HIIT Cardio is where you perform a cardiovascular exercise in intervals, e.g., slow jog for one minute and then a fast run for one minute and you do this for the duration of the workout. The reason that High Intensity Interval Training works better for fat loss is this: When you do a cardio session at the same pace the whole time, your body goes into what is called a steady state. This means that your body has adjusted itself to the speed you are going and tries hard to conserve energy (calories). You will be able to avoid this and burn more calories and FAT by doing the interval training.

If your primary goal is fat loss but to also hold on to and build lean muscle, then lower impact cardio is a must. (see page 163)

**What are the best types of cardio training?** Anything that increases the heart rate for a sustained time is considered good cardio. Running, jogging, walking, playing soccer, rowing and cycling are all great forms of cardio. If you can get to a gym all the better, if not, no problem, try walking and cycling as these are great ways to burn off that unwanted fat. HIIT cardio is best performed with the treadmill, elliptical, rower, stationery bike or stepper. (For more ideas see page 169)

**I've been doing the program for the six weeks and have been amazed by the results, I've lost a lot of flab around my stomach, but I've still not got a six pack, why is this?** Your six pack is still under the remainder of your stomach fat! You need to have very little excess fat covering your abs for them to show, therefore, you need to continue with the program, increase cardio activity and make sure you're sticking to the nutritional plan 100%. Stick to it and you'll see the results in the coming weeks. Remember body fat levels must be reduced to under 10% for your abs to become visible. Purchase a good Body Fat Caliper to monitor your progress and see where your current body fat level is.

**Will too much cardio diminish muscle size?** Yes, more is not always better! You must be careful not to over-train. For those of you wishing to maintain muscular size you must be careful not to do too much when it comes to cardio. Stick to my recommendation earlier. I recommend supplementing with L-Glutamine which will help avoid shrinkage whilst on an intensive training program. See the Supplementation Chapter. (Page 159)

**What will be the first sign that my abs are beginning to show. Will my stomach have slight indentions?** If you currently have a layer of fat around your stomach then the first sign will be a tightening of the midsection as the fat begins to retreat. After time you will begin to see abdominal definition, this will come in the form of 'cuts' or 'ridges'. The clarity of your abdominal muscles will be based on your body fat percentage, the lower your body fat percentage the more definition you will see. For visible definition men require a body fat percentage of less than 10% and women 15%.

**My questions are about EMS (electric muscle stimulation). Do the EMS ab machines work?** These machines were originally designed for athletes who were unable to train due to injury. The idea being to stimulate the muscles to prevent them wasting away rather than improving them. It should be remembered that these devices DO NOT BURN FAT and that is the key to achieving great abs. Abdominal definition will only become visible if your diet is clean, you have a good workout program in place and you perform cardio at least 4 times per week. Some EMS ab devices can help, but only if you have very low body fat levels and almost no fat covering your stomach. My advice would be to stick to traditional exercises coupled with a good diet and exercise program.

**I know the best time to do cardio is before breakfast but the gym I go to for my cardio does not open until 10:30, I wake up about 8:00 am each day and was just wondering if it was ok to consume protein only meals (egg whites) before cardio and still get the desired results?** Protein should be consumed 30 minutes before your session, this is to lessen the risk of muscle catabolism. With your gym opening late, you could do cardio at home or go out for a run.

**I am currently in my 4th week of the training program and am seeing good improvements in tone, however not directly around my abs region. I have been training 3 days a week and keeping to the diet as best as I can. Due to being at university I cannot eat the 5-6 meals a day and often the food I eat is what I can get at the canteen. Do you have advice on this situation and how I can see a bigger improvement in fat loss and flatter abs.** As you often hear throughout the book, diet accounts for as much as 80% of your success. If you cannot stick to a clean diet you will not be making the progress you could be. If you really want abs you cannot afford to stick to the program with 50% commitment, it has to be all or nothing. You must try and adhere to 5-6 smaller sized meals daily. Try and prepare foods and shakes the night before, this will make things much easier. You can then place your meals in food containers ready for the next day. It's also worth investing in a George Foreman Grill, these are fantastic pieces of equipment and an absolute must for anyone at University. I would encourage you to make a bigger commitment to getting your diet on track, once you do, the results will surprise you!

**Just recently I've been feeling rundown. I feel tired and have very little energy to train. I also cannot shake off my sore-throat and cold. Any suggestions?** You're overtraining! Overtraining will make you susceptible to sickness and eventually burnout. You need to take a step back and if need be, have a full week off the gym. Overtraining may also cause symptoms such as insomnia, leading to sleep deprivation, loss of appetite, headaches/migraines, irritability, exhaustion, depression, increases susceptibility to colds and flu and delayed recovery from exercise. So what's the cure? As with most things, prevention is by far the better option and you can do this by making simple changes.

Make small and gradual increases to your exercise and nutrition program over a period of time, avoid jumping in at the deep end. Ensure you get adequate relaxation and sleep, failure to get at least 6 hours per night will cause your immune system to weaken. Try to monitor other stresses in your life, both at home and in your job and make adjustments to suit. Avoid monotonous training, by varying your exercise schedule as much as possible. Do not under any circumstances train when you're ill. You must allow your body to recover first.

If you do find that you're feeling any of the overtraining symptoms above, your first priority is to put your feet up and rest. Anywhere from 3 to 7 days, depending on how severe your symptoms are. During this time forget about exercise, your body MUST be rested. A physical rest, as well as a mental rest. Once symptoms have cleared you can then head back to the gym and gradually implement your routine. You will of course be weak, but full strength and energy will resume after 5-7 days.

It is also important to monitor your diet. Lack of carbs will cause energy loss which will result in getting burned out. As mentioned earlier in the book, it is vitally important to increase carbohydrates on days you exercise.

**Due to my job I often have to eat out at restaurants with clients. What advice would you give me to make better choices when eating out.** Always look for chicken/turkey/fish or lean meat dishes when it comes to eating out. Choose breasts over legs or wings when it comes to poultry. A fillet steak would be preferential to rump, sirloin, T-Bone or flank. Most good restaurants will grill your food, so don't be afraid to ask. Vegetables, salad, potatoes and rice are all good choices too. And don't forget to ask the waiter for some water. Oriental choices when eating out are limited. Chinese foods should ideally be avoided, but preferred options would be stir fry, noodles or dishes containing nuts or beans. With Indian cuisine, basmati rice, noodles or dishes containing pulses such as dhal are fine. And for Italian, pasta, mixed salads with low fat dressings should be your first choices, avoiding anything creamy or cheesy like carbonara.

**Is eating at the likes of McDonalds / Burger King / Subway strictly off limits? Or are there any healthier fast food options I can include in my diet?** Most fast food chains have added healthier options to their menus in the past couple of years in an effort to entice those who are more health conscious, remarkably the likes of McDonalds and Burger King are probably still less fattening than a full curry meal you would find in a restaurant! There are a few options that you can have on occasion, but as always, preparing your own foods should always be your first choice.

There are a few basic rules you should keep in mind when trying to pick healthier fast food options. Good options include, the smallest size of burger, grilled chicken sandwiches or salads, low-fat dressings and sauces (or none at all) and either diet soft drinks or water. Below are the best options available from some of the more recognised fast food chains.

| Burger King® | Calories | Fat | Protein | Carbs |
|---|---|---|---|---|
| BK Broiler Chicken Sandwich | 267 | 8 | 22 | 25 |
| Frozen Yogurt (Vanilla) | 120 | 3 | 0 | 20 |
| Salad Chunky Chicken | 142 | 4 | 20 | 8 |
| Side Salad | 25 | 0 | 0 | 5 |

| McDonald's® | Calories | Fat | Protein | Carbs |
|---|---|---|---|---|
| English Muffin | 140 | 2 | 0 | 25 |
| Chicken McGrill no/mayo | 340 | 7 | 26 | 45 |
| Hamburger | 280 | 10 | 12 | 35 |

| Subway® | Calories | Fat | Protein | Carbs |
|---|---|---|---|---|
| *All subs on Wholewheat* | | | | |
| 6" Veggie Delite | 250 | 2.5 | 11 | 37 |
| 6" Veg Shammi | 254 | 3.0 | 10 | 39 |
| 6" Veggie Patty | 250 | 2.5 | 10 | 39 |
| 6" Paneer Tikka | 300 | 7.0 | 18 | 40 |
| 6" Honey, Mustard, Turkey | 275 | 3.5 | 22 | 42 |
| 6" Chicken/Ham Sub | 261 | 4.5 | 17 | 39 |
| 6" Roast Beef | 264 | 4.5 | 18 | 39 |
| 6" Roast Chicken | 311 | 4.0 | 25 | 40 |
| 6" Chicken Tikka | 250 | 4.0 | 23 | 40 |
| 6" Turkey Sub | 254 | 3.5 | 16 | 39 |

**If I accidentally skip a cardio and/or weightlifting session (including abs), should I workout harder and add an additional workout session the day after? Or, should I continue as if I didn't skip one (what do you recommend)?** It is important not to miss a session, therefore you should try to make it up either the day after or sometime later in the week. Missing a session and leaving it will just put you behind with making progress, so try to keep up the momentum and include it sometime during the week.

**I thought in school I was taught that 1 pound = 1 pound. Now I hear people saying that muscle weights more than fat. This mathematically doesn't make sense to me. If you have one pound of fat and 1 pound of muscle and weigh them both, they will both weigh 1 pound. So how does muscle weigh more than fat if on a scale they should both theoretically weigh the same?** Correct, one pound of muscle weighs one pound. One pound of fat also weighs one pound. They both weigh the same. However, muscle is denser than fat, so one pound of muscle will take up less space than one pound of fat.

**How do I know when HIIT cardio is intense enough?** The chances are you'll be sweating by the end! When you run during the intensive part of the workout, you should be doing so at about 85-90% of your maximum effort. The jogging part should be reduced to about 60-75% of your maximum, which will allow you to get your breath back.

How much does one's age factor into developing six pack abs? I understand as one ages; the metabolism rate slows, the body begins to gain weight and other natural ageing processes begin. I think the diet routine is probably the most difficult to maintain for maximum results in obtaining a great set of abs. What is your opinion about the correlation between age and the ability to develop (to see) the abdominal region?

Age can play a factor in developing six pack abs. You nailed it when you mentioned that the body's metabolism slows down and the body gains weight as you get older, you may also become less active, which may also lead to weight gain. However, age is a double edged sword. If you have stayed in shape, watched your diet and trained your whole life, it's going to be a lot easier for you to get a tight set of abs than it would be for someone who hasn't trained in years. For example, I know some guys that are well into their 40's and 50's and have totally ripped physiques and abs. Go online and search a guy called Clarence Bass who is 70 years old, he exemplifies perfect conditioning in ones later years, he is completely ripped. Guys like this have trained for years though, and they know their body like the back of their hand. They have muscle maturity, experience, and knowledge. They know exactly how long it takes them to get ripped, what they need to eat, what foods work best for their body, how much cardio they need to do, and how often they need to train. It's amazing. But it does come down to real hard work and absolute dedication to maintain great shape in your later years. At whatever age you're at, if you can lose enough body fat around your midsection, then your abs will become visible. It's not as easy as it sounds, but it's possible.

**What is the best thing I can snack on? I have just quit smoking and am finding it hard not to eat!**

First let me congratulate you! You've made a huge step towards a better and healthier life. Quitting smoking is no easy feat. Because smoking is a form of addiction, 80 percent of smokers who quit usually experience some withdrawal symptoms. These may include increased appetite. The symptoms may be intense for two or three days, but within 10 to 30 days after quitting, most subside. Because smoking creates both physical and psychological dependency someone tries to find other alternatives providing the same pleasurable sensation tobacco may offer, such as cravings for junk food. In addition to this, when you quit smoking you have an elevated appetite, as Nicotine is a well-known appetite suppressor. But if you do this all the time you will gain dozens of pounds in no time. Therefore, you should adapt a healthy diet that has a good balance of carbohydrates, proteins and some good fats. When it gets particularly hard with cravings I would suggest snacking on nuts and seeds. Flavored Rice Cakes can also be good at controlling those cravings. Salads, green veggies are equally just as good. A fantastic low fat, low calorie snack would be **Yellow Split Pea Dhal**. Here's the recipe which makes 8 small portions (*103 calories and 16g carbs, 3.5g protein each serving*).

Caution - it's got a bit of a kick! This easy dhal recipe is very low in fat and is also low-calorie.

*Ingredients:*
1 cup yellow split peas, uncooked, 2 cups water or vegetable broth, 1 tsp turmeric, ¼ tsp cayenne, ½ tsp salt, 1 tbsp margarine, 1 onion, diced, 1 ½ tsp cumin, whole seeds or ground, 2 whole cloves, dash pepper, to taste

*Preparation:*

In a large pot, place the peas and water or vegetable broth, and bring to a slow simmer. Add the turmeric, cayenne and salt, and cover. Allow to cook for at least 20 minutes, stirring occasionally.

In a large skillet or frying pan, heat the onion, cumin and clove in the margarine. Cook for 4 to 6 minutes, until onion is soft. Add the onion and spices to the split peas, and allow to simmer for at least 5 more minutes.

| Nutritional Info. | Calories | Fat | Protein | Carbs |
|---|---|---|---|---|
| Yellow Split Pea Dhal | 103 | 4.5 | 6.5 | 16 |

# Conversions

## Weight/Mass

1 kg = 2.2 pounds

500 grams = 1.1 pounds

1 pound = 0.45 kg

4 oz = 113 grams

## Consumption

1 gallon = 4.5 Liters

## Length

1 inch = 2.5 cm

1 yard = 0.9 metres

1 kilometer = 0.6 miles

1 foot = 30 centimeters

## Macronutrients

1 gram of protein = 4 Calories

1 gram of carbs = 4 Calories

1 gram of fat = 9 Calories

# Bollywood Abs

## by NEIL FROST

*Photography by:*
BIG Picture UK

*Cover Model:* Saurabh Ram Lubhaya
*Other Models:* Abhishek Das, Panos Kalafolias, Alon Gabbay